# Nursing Care Planning Guides
## Set 2
### Second Edition

**Margo Creighton Neal, RN, MN**
VICE PRESIDENT, WILLIAMS & WILKINS

**Patricia Feltz Cohen, RN, MA, EdM**
CONSULTANT, HUNTINGTON BEACH, CA

**Phyllis Gorney Cooper, RN, MN**
CONSULTANT, LOS ANGELES, CA

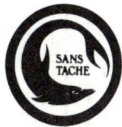

WILLIAMS & WILKINS
Baltimore • London • Los Angeles • Sydney

*Printed in the United States of America*

**Library of Congress Cataloging in Publication Data**

Main entry under title:
Nursing care planning guides, set 2, 2nd Ed.

    1. Nursing—Handbooks, manuals, etc.  2. Nursing—Planning—Handbooks, manuals, etc.  I. Neal, Margo Creighton, 1935–    , joint author.  II. Cohen, Patricia Feltz, 1932–    , joint author.  III. Cooper, Phyllis Gorney, 1946–    , joint author. IV. Title. [DNLM: 1. Patient care planning—Handbooks.  2. Nursing care—Handbooks.  WY100 N342n]
RT51.N37    1981    610.73    80-23377
ISBN 0-683-09520-X

    86  87  88  89    10  9  8  7  6  5  4

# PREFACE

This revised edition of Nursing Care Planning Guides Set 2 updates the 50 topics contained in its pages.

Many changes have occurred in nursing since the first edition was printed in 1975. The basic nursing process, however, has remained the same and the main focus of this work is, like its predecessor, to help nurses use nursing process to plan individualized care for their patients/clients.

This revised edition contains all goals and objectives in terms of patient behaviors or expected outcomes of care. The categories of patient problems have been revised to reflect the growing use of nursing diagnoses, and the reference lists have been updated.

In this edition, we attempted to avoid stereotyping the nurse as "she" and the patient as "he" by using "s/he" in lieu of she/he. However, the English language has not yet produced a combination form for masculine and feminine pronouns, thus you will note some referral to the patient in the masculine form only.

Margo C. Neal
Patricia F. Cohen
Phyllis G. Cooper

# FOREWORD

Nursing process is the essence of nursing. This Set of Nursing Care Planning Guides can help nurses use nursing process to plan individualized patient care and transfer the data into written nursing care plans.

Each of these Nursing Care Planning Guides is written in the format of a nursing care plan and contains all the basic components: long term goals, areas of patient problems, patient outcomes, and nursing actions.

It is expected that a nurse will assess the "specific considerations" category (eg. cardiopulmonary function) and if there is a problem, define it specifically (eg. decreased cardiac output), then select a patient outcome and nursing actions from those suggested in the Guide. Not all of the suggested outcomes and actions will be appropriate for each patient.

Additional information is also provided for the nurses' own use: definition and general considerations of the condition, nursing responsibilities, and recommended references.

To use these Guides most efficiently, scan the Table of Contents. Note that this Set is comprised of three sections: A) med-surg conditions; B) patient behaviors; and C) supplementary information. You may wish to consult more than one Guide per patient. For example, a patient is admitted with extensive burns. Refer to #2:05, "The Patient with Burns: Critical-Acute Phase," and #2:28, "The Burn Patient: Common Behaviors."

This Set is also cross-referenced to three additional sets of Nursing Care Planning Guides, Sets 2, 3, and 4. For detailed information on each condition, consult med-surg texts.

Nursing Care Planning Guides should be used as guidelines and ready-references only, not as standard care plans. To use them as the latter would negate individual differences in patients, thus contradicting the original purpose of care plans . . . i.e. individualized patient care.

# Set No. 2
## TABLE OF CONTENTS

# The Patient with Alcoholism

**Definition:** A physiological dependence (addiction) on alcohol as a result of excessive use.

**LONG TERM GOAL:** The patient will be able to recognize and accept his addiction and to develop situational supports and coping mechanisms that reflect adaptation to a life style without alcohol.

## General Considerations:

— In general hospitals, a patient with alcoholism is often admitted with another diagnosis which may or may not be related to use of alcohol. Excessive use can cause many physical problems such as: gastritis, chronic diarrhea, vitamin and nutritional deficiencies, disorders of neurological and cardiac systems, pancreatitis, fatty liver, cirrhosis, hypoglycemia.

— The **cause** of alcoholism is not known, but it seems to be affected by: (1) *social factors* (customs, attitudes towards drinking; amount of stress and tension in the community), and (2) the individual's *personality traits* (tend to be generally uneasy and dissatisfied with life; tend to excesses in areas such as work, sex, recreation; low frustration tolerance; dependence on others; poor ability to cope with stress).

— Alcohol depresses higher cortical functions, acts as a disinhibitor and tranquilizer and serves to reduce anxiety rapidly; excessive drinking is often the way a person copes with anxiety.

— Alcohol addiction often creates behavioral responses that are considered erratic, irresponsible, destructive. It may create a situation where the alcohol need is dominant and the purpose of living is to maintain alcohol intake.

— The **severity of withdrawal** symptoms is the direct result of the increased levels of acetaldehyde and decreased magnesium levels in the blood (breakdown products of alcohol).

— **General treatment measures** include vitamin and nutritional therapy, use of sedatives, tranquilizers, and/or Antabuse.

— **Preventive measures** include helping the patient learn (1) to tolerate psychological stress; (2) to do advance planning for anticipated painful events (surgery, separation from a loved one); and (3) to reduce social isolation.

— **Nursing responsibilities** include adequate treatment and maintenance of life functions during withdrawal, as well as teaching and support of preventative measures in those predisposed to alcoholism.

## Specific Considerations, Potential Patient Outcomes, and Nursing Actions:

1) Maintenance of Body Functioning During

The patient will withdraw from the alcohol free of the complications of dehydration, electrolyte imbalance, nutritional imbalance; will verbally recognize and discuss his alcoholism as the cause of the withdrawal:

— know that the severity of withdrawal symptoms is related to the length & extent of drinking preceding the withdrawal period;

| Withdrawal | — complete cessation of use of alcohol is not necessary for the development of withdrawal symptoms; the beginning of withdrawal can be a reflection of diminished use in those who have developed a high tolerance and physical dependence; observe for withdrawal symptoms as early as 8 hours after cessation of drinking; |
|---|---|
| | — withdrawal is a progressive process and involves four stages: |

Stage I — 8 hours + after cessation: symptoms include mild tremors, nausea, nervousness, tachycardia, increased blood pressure, & diaphoresis.

Stage II — symptoms include gross tremors, nervousness & hyperactivity, insomnia, anorexia, general weakness, disorientation, illusions, nightmares; auditory & visual hallucinations begin.

Stage III — 12-48 hours after cessation: symptoms include all those of Stages I and II, as well as severe hallucinations & grand mal seizures.

Stage IV — occurs 3-5 days after cessation: symptoms include initial & continuing DTs (delirium tremens) which are characterized by confusion, severe psychomotor activity, agitation, sleeplessness, hallucinations, & uncontrolled & unexplained tachycardia at onset.

— control symptoms via PRN medication; take vital signs Q2H & report elevated ones to doctor;

— if pt. is agitated, confused, etc., stay with him; reassure that current symptoms are only result of his body responding to alcohol use, & that they are temporary; tell him he will regain control; use restraints only if absolutely necessary;

— deal with hallucinations by reinforcing reality; speak to pt. slowly in a calm voice; provide a quiet environment; stay with pt. until the frightening symptoms have decreased;

— ensure a daily fluid intake of at least 2500 cc's orally (unless contraindicated; check with Dr.); offer favorite juices Q2H during waking hours; prevent excessive coffee or tea intake;

— identify pt.'s food preferences; provide frequent small feedings or in-between meal snacks of high-protein foods; involve pt. in food-related planning; give multivitamin & mineral supplements as ordered;

— provide physical care advocated for additional diseases/conditions pt. may have;

— keep pt. ambulatory as much as possible; if necessary, walk with pt. several times a day; help to bathroom, rather than providing bed pan or urinal.

2) Psychosocial Adjustment (to Life without Alcohol) — The patient will discuss and develop the use of coping mechanism other than alcohol to deal with the stress and strain of daily life:

— sit & visit with pt. at least twice daily; your presence will say s/he is not being rejected for any behavior;

— discuss your observations of pt.'s behavior with him, helping him develop insight re: its relation with alcohol intake;

— in an accepting, non-judgmental way, discuss pt.'s use of alcohol with him; provide information as he wants and asks for it; seek help of a psychiatric nurse or mental health specialist if you cannot do this;

— recognize & share with pt. that a lifestyle without alcohol is a major loss to him (see NCPG #1:31, "Response to Loss. . ."); anticipate what this may mean & help him plan adaptive ways to compensate for the loss;

— do not punish or reprimand pt. for failures or nonresponse to your suggestions/interventions; (punishment serves only to give pt. fuel for continuing to deal with failure or rejection by drinking) ignore it, but do praise *any* positive responses;

— have pt. make decisions about daily care in hospital; involve him in some type of occupational therapy, anything in which he can achieve some measure of success (helps increase self-confidence and self-esteem);

— provide opportunities to decrease social isolation & improve social skills (meal times, pt. groups, recreation periods); calmly, gently, point out unacceptable behavior such as manipulative ones (see NCPG #1:20, "The Patient Displaying Manipulation"); reinforce positive social behaviors (e.g. initiating friendly conversations); praise all efforts at participation in activities;

— if pt. on Antabuse therapy, read literature & then explain effects that develop with ingestion of alcohol (severe nausea & vomiting, flushed face, rapid pulse and respirations, drop in BP);

— arrange for pt. & family to attend group counseling sessions, if available in hospital, to discuss feelings, problems, changing behaviors, pressures, sources of support, etc.;

— discuss AA with pt.; offer to arrange for a member to come & see pt. & encourage him to accept; provide information about other types of therapy available, e.g. local mental health clinics.

3) Functional, Situational Support Systems

The patient will accept the support of others; will discuss with them how they can help him live without alcohol:

— hold weekly health team conferences to discuss aspects of alcoholism, share feelings & responses to caring for an alcoholic pt., & to coordinate care; explain that it is normal for staff to feel frustrated (angry, guilty, rejecting, anxious) when caring for alcoholic pts.; staff often feel they have failed if a pt. is readmitted in an alcoholic state after they had discharged him "improved"; include a psych. nurse or other mental health specialist;

— request inservice education programs, films, literature, etc. on alcoholism;

— permit family to express their anger at pt.'s exacerbations; listen to & support them; put family in touch with a community group where consistent support & help are available, e.g. Al Anon (family group of AA);

— invite a member of AA &/or Al Anon to a staff conference to share their aims, approaches, etc., or go to a meeting with a colleague.

**Discharge Planning and Teaching Objectives/Outcomes**

1. (Patient/Family/Significant Other) Has a contact with Alcoholics Anonymous, Al Anon and/or other community mental health group.
2) Verbalizes an understanding of and expects to participate in a daily program of balanced food and fluid intake, rest, exercise, and recreation.
3) Can state the actions and side effects of current medications; has an adequate supply to take with him.
4) Has at least one plan to help decrease social isolation and strengthen new behaviors.

**Recommended References**

"Alcoholism" (and other publications). National Council on Alcoholism, Inc., 2 Park Avenue, New York, NY 10016.

"Assessing Alcoholic Patients," by E. Heinemann and N. Estes. *American Journal of Nursing*, May 1976:785–789.

"Helping the Alcoholic Cope With . . . Sobriety," by Mary Ann Boyson. *RN*, July 1975:37.

"Maternal Alcoholism and the Fetal Alcohol Syndrome," by Barbara Luke. *American Journal of Nursing*, December 1977:1924–1926.

"Rehabilitating the Problem Drinker," by J. Carroll and M. Synigal. *Nursing Digest*, Fall, 1976:44–46.

"Rehabilitation for Alcoholics," by Joyce Ditzler. *American Journal of Nursing*, November 1976:1772–1774.

"Responses to Loss: the Grief and Mourning Process." NCP Guide #1:31, 2nd ed., Nurseco, 1980.

"The Alcoholic Surgical Patient," Nursing Grand Rounds, *Nursing '77*, May 1977:56–61.

"The Value of Life," Nursing Grand Rounds, *Nursing '79*, July 1979:30–37.

# The Patient with Asthma

**Definition:**   A reversible, obstructive condition of the small bronchioles, accompanied by an audible wheeze, more pronounced on expiration than inspiration.

**LONG TERM GOAL:**   The patient will regain a steady level of respiratory health through a regimen of rest, exercise, nutrition, and avoidance of precipitants to an asthmatic attack.

## General Considerations:
— Asthma is not a disease, but **a condition initiated by** an antigen-antibody reaction that releases histamine and a slow-reacting substance of anaphylaxis. This results in dilated blood vessels, production of excess mucus, edema, and contraction of the small muscles in the airways. Subsequent reactions include wheezing, bronchospasm, a decrease in lung ventilation, and an alteration in exchange of respiratory gases.
— **Precipitants** to an attack may be extrinsic or intrinsic:
   *extrinsic:* allergies to pollens, dust, foods, smoke, cold air, feathers, mold spores, stress;
   *intrinsic:* abnormalities in respiratory tract, infected tracheo-bronchial lymph nodes, pulmonary infections, emotional stress.
— **Onset** of an attack is usually sudden, with a cough and tightness in chest, followed by slow, laborious wheezing; may last from ½-several hours, then will finally subside; patient may be perspiring, cold, have a weak pulse, fever, pain, N/V or diarrhea; attacks are exhausting but rarely fatal except in *status asthmaticus:* a series of repeated episodes which are life threatening. Once started, attacks may continue as "asthma habit."
— Asthma appears to have a hereditary tendency in ⅔'s of all cases; 50% of hay fever attacks end as asthma.
— Treatment is symptomatic for an acute attack; long term care involves measures to control the precipitants.
— **Nursing responsibilities** include helping to relieve the acute distress, and teaching a health maintenance regimen.

## Specific Considerations, Potential Patient Outcomes, and Nursing Actions:
1) Respiratory   Patient will maintain a patent airway; will resume a normal breathing pattern; will liquefy and raise mucus:
   Distress
   — observe & chart rate & character of respirations, temperature, pulse, color, diaphoresis, cough, amount & appearance of expectorated sputum;
   — position pt. in a comfortable sitting position, eg. high Fowler's, in a chair, on side of bed, leaning on a pillow on an overbed table, with feet on chair;

— give $O_2$ to relieve cyanosis & anoxia; use a mist tent PRN to increase humidity & liquefy secretions;
— increase oral intake to 3-4000 cc's/day, unless contraindicated; check with Dr.; keep fluids at bedside (water & pt.'s choices);
— keep an ample supply of tissues & disposal bag at bedside;
— keep endotracheal tubes, laryngoscope, & tracheostomy equipment at bedside for emergency use;
— teach pt. to use diaphragm rather than just lungs to pull in & expel deep breaths of air when s/he first feels a tightening sensation in chest;
— read NCPG #3:40, "Acid-Base Balance."

2) Anxiety and Fear

The patient will use anxiety-reducing techniques to lower anxiety level; will express the feelings s/he is experiencing:

— stay with pt. during an acute attack; use physical contact you deem appropriate to assure pt. you are there to help; allow family/significant other to stay if pt. wishes;
— ask pt. to close eyes & concentrate on visualizing himself breathing calmly & efficiently; repeat several times, checking pt.'s respirations for any change; explain that the bronchi are *temporarily* in spasm, & will soon begin to relax;
— decrease pt.'s "closed-in" feeling by keeping curtains & doors open, bed clothes loose, etc.;
— reduce stimuli by keeping questions to pt. at a minimum, room quiet, lights dimmed, noise reduced (will help pt. relax & rest);
— read NCPGs #1:22 & 1:28, "Anxiety" & "Fear";
— when acute phase is over, ensure that pt. is allowed to sleep *undisturbed.*

3) Medications

The patient experiences symptomatic relief via medications; verbalizes actions, side effects of prescribed medications:
— see NCPG #2:36, "Drugs: Asthma";
— assess pt. & family's knowledge of drugs given & teach PRN;
— encourage to take only prescribed medications after discharge.

4) Prevention of Complications and Recurrences

The patient can identify factors precipitating an attack, and has alternatives for avoiding them as much as possible; the patient will be free of secondary infections:
— do attacks seem to be triggered by intrinsic or extrinsic factors? work with pt. & family to devise ways to avoid/alter these as much as possible, including fatigue, chilling, exposure to others who have a URI, stressful experiences;

— teach pt. to call Dr. at first sign of a cold or change in color of sputum;
— assess pt.'s knowledge of a balanced program of rest, exercise, & nutrition; correct & teach PRN; pt. should exercise regularly, but stop short of fatigue; ensure pt. has regular rest periods 1-2 times daily.

## Discharge Planning and Teaching Objectives/Outcomes

1) (Patient/Family/Significant Other) Can identify factors which precipitate an attack, and knows steps to take to avoid these factors.
2) Knows what steps to take at signs of an impending attack.
3) Knows how to administer injections and/or aerosol inhalations at home.
4) Knows signs and symptoms of impending respiratory infection, including changes in sputum, and to seek medical assistance.
5) Has a written list of medications, including dosage, actions and possible side effects for each one.
6) Has developed a balanced program of nutrition, rest, and exercise.

**Recommended References**

"Acid-Base Balance." NCP Guide #3:40, Nurseco, 1977.

"Drugs: Asthma." NCP Guide #2:36, 2nd Ed., Nurseco, 1980.

"Responses to Loss: the Grief and Mourning Process." NCP Guide # 1:31, 2nd Ed., Nurseco, 1980.

"The Patient Experiencing Fear." NCP Guide #1:28, 2nd Ed., Nurseco, 1980.

"The Patient Experiencing Anxiety." NCP Guide #1:22, 2nd Ed., Nurseco, 1980.

## The Patient for Bladder Retraining

**LONG TERM GOAL:** The patient re-establishes partial to full control of bladder and a satisfactory pattern of elimination without retention or overflow; the patient will regain the best possible function of the urinary tract without infection or concomitant complications, such as skin breakdown; the patient will experience an increase in self-esteem, dignity and a measure of independence.

### General Considerations:
— **Types:** Involuntary loss of urine may be *stress* incontinence (when coughing, laughing, sneezing, straining at BM, etc.), *urge* incontinence (voiding upon a sudden urge produced by spasm of irritated bladder walls), or *neurogenic* incontinence (no sensation, no desire to void).
— **Causes:** any acute, prolonged or recurrent urinary tract infection, a loss of muscle tone or sensation (related to childbirth trauma, aging, degenerative diseases, a stroke, a malignancy or a spinal cord lesion or injury), a loss of normal functioning position and schedule (related to prolonged bedrest, emotional depression, physical confinement, etc.), or a loss of control in the cerebrum (related to arteriosclerosis, a tumor or severe disorientation).
— Urinary incontinence often produces social and psychological problems. The patient feels embarrassed, ashamed, guilty, anxious, depressed and helpless. Often they become socially isolated and withdrawn.
— **Treatment** may include: weight reduction if necessary, limitation of alcohol intake, pelvic exercises, drug therapy, bladder retraining and sometimes surgery. Operations may be correction of urethral stenosis, a Marshall-Marchetti-Krantz to correct the urethrovesical angle, A&P colporrhapy, surgical implantation of an artificial sphincter, or other procedure.
— **Successful bladder retraining** programs begin with an *assessment* of the patient's general physical and mental condition; the urological tract function; the cause, length of time and degree of incontinence, and the anticipated cooperation of the patient and family in the program. *Diagnostic tests* include cystoscopy, IV pyelogram, cystometric & uroflometric studies, culture & sensitivity studies. The program is tailored to the individual patient's needs, a consent to participate is obtained, and the health team collaborates to implement the plan.

### Specific Considerations, Potential Patient Outcomes, and Nursing Actions:
1) Urine Quality & Quantity  The patient's urine maintains a normal pH, specific gravity, volume and composition; the formation of calculi and bacterial growth is retarded or prevented:
   — have the pt. drink 2000-2500 ml. of fluid each day during waking hours, preferably before the evening meal;
   — give 6-8 oz. cranberry or prune juice daily to acidify the urine;
   — avoid unusual amounts of orange juice which helps produce alkalinity;

— if not otherwise contraindicated, coffee, tea & beer may stimulate micturition;
— know that a low calcium diet (1 gm. per day) to reduce chances of stones may be ordered;
— record intake & output accurately, until adequacy is assured;
— record urine specific gravity once daily (afternoon specimen); order a urinalysis at least once weekly;
— give medications as ordered (urinary antiseptics, antispasmodics & antibiotics); note side effects & record pt. response.

**2) Voiding Procedure**

The patient will restore normal voiding patterns; the patient's muscle tone will improve, especially bladder detrusor fibers and the internal and external sphincters; retention with overflow will be prevented; at least partial bladder control will be restored:

— begin with a day & night voiding schedule of every 1 to 2 hours; keep a regular & consistent pattern for at least two days; then increase the intervals by half hour increments every few days until four hour intervals between voiding are attained (for some pts., a 1-2 hrs. voiding pattern may remain necessary); except when sleeping, pt. should not be asked to hold his urine more than four hours; waking the pt. once each night to void is often desirable;
— help initiate micturition: have the pt. take a long, slow deep breath, then tighten abdominal and pelvic muscles, then relax; a measured amt. of warm water poured over the vulva or penis may be helpful; the sound of running water sometimes helps;
— measure the initial amt. voided; then press on the lower abdomen over the bladder to enable expression of remaining urine (Crede's Method of manual expression); measure this amt. voided; pts. with neurogenic bladder may be taught this procedure for continuing use;
— avoid the use of an indwelling or intermittent catheter unless necessary for medical reasons or as a last resort to prevent retention & potential kidney damage; if used, plan for periodic clamping & unclamping of the catheter in order to maintain as much normal bladder size & muscle tone as possible; tidal drainage methods occasionally may be used to develop automatic bladder control;
— have pt. practice alternate periods of contraction & relaxation of pubococcygeal muscles to develop improved muscle tone & sphincter control; these "Kegel" exercises should be done QID;
— use sanitary pads, undergarments with reinforced panels, & terrycloth or "Chux" type bedpads for stress incontinence or dribbling; never use diapers unless the pt. is severely disoriented or comatose & bladder retraining cannot be accomplished; external (condom over penis) drainage tubing is often used for male patients.

**Discharge Planning and Teaching Objectives/Outcomes**

1) (Patient/Family/Significant Other) Can state in their own words the basic cause of incontinence, the plan for retraining the bladder and what the patient's part in the program is, initially, and at home.

2) Can verbalize indications for seeking prompt medical attention (i.e. signs of infection, medication intolerance of side effects, recurrence of retention with overflow, burning or itching while voiding, etc.).

**Recommended References**

"Assessing Urinary Incontinence In Women," by Priscilla Butts. *Nursing 79*, March 1979:72–74.

"Catheters: Indwelling Urethral." *NCP Guide* #2:39, Nurseco, 2nd Ed., 1980.

# The Patient for Bowel Retraining

**LONG TERM GOAL:**    The patient re-establishes good bowel function and a satisfactory pattern of evacuation without dependence on harsh laxatives.

## General Considerations:
— A bowel retraining program is recommended for patients with chronic elimination problems of constipation or fecal incontinence.
— **Constipation exists:** (1) when the consistency of the feces is too hard for elimination without pain; (2) when the amount of feces is too small and a portion remains in the rectum after defecation; or (3) when the length of time between eliminations is abnormally long for that individual.
— **Fecal incontinence exists** when elimination occurs involuntarily and may be a sign of: (1) loss of sphincter control, or (2) impaction.
— **Treatment** for the improvement of bowel function includes:
  • a comprehensive assessment of contributing factors;
  • the correction of faulty elimination habits;
  • improvement of the general health;
  • intake of a proper diet and fluid volume;
  • regular exercise; and, usually,
  • bulk-forming and stool-softening medications.

## Specific Considerations, Potential Patient Outcomes, and Nursing Actions:
1) Assessment of    The causes and contributing factors for the chronic elimination problem will be identified; a data base for determination of an
   Problem           appropriate bowel retraining will be provided:
   — obtain from the pt. & his family a dietary history, listing foods & fluids that have caused constipation, flatus or gastric distress; list those foods & fluids that have produced a loose stool for the pt; evaluate the amount of roughage foods usually consumed;
   — record the pt.'s usual (when well) & present bowel patterns; question frequency, amount, consistency, & time of day that elimination most often occurs; identify pt.'s own signs of a full bowel (loss of appetite? headache? abdominal fullness or pain? restlessness?); identify environmental stimuli to evacuation or personal habits (cup of coffee? smoking? reading? privacy? personal bathroom? glass of hot water with a juice of lemon?);
   — learn the pattern of exercise, kind & amount, past & present;

— determine the usage of laxatives & enemas: kind, amount, frequency; what other medications are ingested which may cause constipation (codeine? sedatives? etc.);
— what other factors may be contributing to constipation in this pt.? (hemorrhoids? anal fissure or fistula? growth of tumor? recent surgery? depression, senility and deterioration?);
— examine rectum for impaction & record results.

2) Habit Formation The patient's pattern of elimination will be established with acceptable regularity and without repeated accidents:
— based on the data assessed above, plan to correct, eliminate or modify all factors contributing to constipation or incontinence;
— with the pt./family, determine a suitable time daily to attempt defecation; consider, but do not be bound to, time of day formerly used, if factors indicate a new time is presently desirable; encourage the pt. to notify you of any urge to defecate at any other time of the day & be prompt to take advantage of natural urges;
— reproduce helpful environmental stimuli that have been successful (i.e. a warm bathroom or commode seat, absolute privacy, coffee, tea or other hot liquid, reading material, etc.);
— position pt. in a sitting position, out of bed, whenever possible;
— provide a foot stool, so the pt. can push against it; also it helps maintain a slight knee-chest position known to facilitate a natural bowel movement; bedfast patients should bend their knees, if able, & press their heels against the bed; raise this pt. to as nearly upright a position as condition permits;
— using abdominal breathing, have the pt. take three, long, slow deep breaths, then tighten abdominal muscles, bear down & push;
— if the pt. is unable to defecate in ten minutes, have him return to bed & rest in a left side-lying position;
— a glycerin or biscodyl (Dulcolax) suppository may be inserted rectally; it should be retained for 15-20 min., then another attempt to eliminate is made;
— if still no results, have the pt. try at other times of the day (after meals or exercise or physical therapy);
— if no results for two days, palpate lower abdomen for a mass in the descending colon or examine rectum for an impaction;
— digital evacuation of lower rectum may be necessary, but a low, oil retention enema may also be tried;
— large amounts of fluid enemas should not be given because they unnecessarily distend the colon and delay bowel retraining.

3) Diet and Fluids   The patient will have normal gastric activity facilitated and a soft, solid stool formed, given appropriate diet and fluids:
  — based on assessment data & a consultation with a dietician, plan to eliminate foods which cause constipation or flatus for this pt.;
  — plan to include in the diet bulk-forming roughage foods such as bran or whole wheat cereals and breads; broccoli, cabbage, spinach, okra, cauliflower, tomatoes, lettuce, celery, apples, oranges, grapes, figs, prunes, & raisins;
  — fresh vegetables & fruits are desirable; they may be shredded or chopped finely for those with chewing problems;
  — ensure an adequate (2000-2500 cc) fluid intake daily;
  — give prune juice, 4-8 oz. at bedtime nightly, or about 8-10 hrs. before the planned time for defecation;
  — upon arising, give pt. a 6 oz. glass of very warm water, mixed with 2 tablespoons lemon juice & 2 tablespoons of honey (which has a slight laxative effect).

4) Supplemental   The patient will re-establish an optimum level of health and activity with as nearly normal a bowel pattern as possible:
   Aids
  — plan for regular daily exercise, especially walking, deep-breathing & abdominal muscle setting exercise;
  — help the pt. maintain own weight within desirable limits, suggesting nutritional supplements as needed;
  — bulk-forming, water absorbing, stool softening agents may be beneficial; psyllium hydrophilic mucilloid (Metamucil) and dioctyl sodium sulfosuccinate (Colace, Doxinate, others) are popular & have proven helpful;
  — avoid use of irritant laxatives (including saline and oil types); side-effects are harmful;
  — digital stimulation or glycerin suppositories may be needed on a long-term basis, especially for the seriously deteriorated patient.

## Discharge Planning and Teaching Objectives/Outcomes

1) (Patient/Family/Significant Other) Can verbalize a basic knowledge and understanding of the bowel retraining program and its various aspects (habit formation, diet, fluids, exercises, what to avoid, etc.).
2) Understands and can state indications for seeking medical attention (i.e. signs of infection, diarrhea, or changing bowel habits, bleeding, etc.)

**Recommended References**

"Bowel Program for Institutionalized Adults," by Marjorie Habeeb and Mina Kallstrom. *American Journal of Nursing,* April 1976:606–608.
"More Fiber-Less Constipation," by Linda Bass. *American Journal of Nursing,* February 1977:254,255.

# The Patient with Burns: Critical-Acute Phase

**Definition:** Burns are injuries to tissues caused by thermal (flame and/or liquid), radioactive, and/or electric agents. The mechanism of injury is the denaturation of protein which results in cell injury or death.

**LONG TERM GOAL:** The patient will recover from the burn without loss of function of any body part; the patient will recover maximum use of the body part.

**General Considerations:**
— **Classification:** a burn is classified according to depth of injury and extent of body surface involved:
  • *1st degree:* partial thickness burn, generally limited to the outer layer of epidermis; characterized by redness, increased warmth, pain and tenderness; no blisters or systemic involvement occurs. Treatment is generally focused on relief of symptoms. Healing occurs within 1 to 2 weeks and there is no scarring.
  • *2nd degree:* partial thickness burn involving total destruction of the epidermis and partial destruction of the dermis; characterized by redness, formation of blisters, edema and pain; systemic involvement occurs when infection and/or trauma is present during the burn wound healing. Healing is by spontaneous epithelial regeneration and treatment is directed towards the support of this process and the prevention of infection. Healing takes several weeks to months.
  • *3rd degree:* full-thickness burn involving total destruction of the epidermis and dermis; characterized by lack of pain (nerve endings are destroyed), edema (due to increased capillary permeability); area appears from waxy white to brown. Healing usually takes months and intensive treatment is necessary since epithelial regeneration does not occur.
  • *4th degree:* full thickness burn involving destruction of the epidermis, dermis, fat, muscle and bone; characterized by lack of pain, edema, eschar (leathery type cover due to surface dehydration); area appears black and depressed. Healing takes months, intensive treatment is necessary and since epithelial regeneration does not occur, grafting is required.
— **Pathophysiological effect** of 2nd, 3rd and 4th degree burns:
  • immediate alterations of the capillary permeability causing edema;
  • hemoconcentration of the blood, a rise in hematocrit level;
  • fluid shifts are rapid and occur readily within first 8 hours; thus, without proper treatment, shock may result; occur at a slower rate 2-3 days post-injury and after 5 days or more, the shift reverses and fluid returns to the vascular compartments;
  • hyperkalemia, due to destruction of tissues;
  • catabolism, causing major loss of potassium and nitrogen.

— **Severity of injury affected by:**
  - age of patient (relates to the difference in amount of surface area and character of skin);
  - causative agent and duration of exposure;
  - level of adaptive coping prior to injury (emotional status);
  - location of injury (relates to areas that are susceptible to greater degrees of impairment, e.g. hands, feet, or can cause systemic involvement, e.g. neck, nasal passages);
  - presence of other pathological conditions (relates to the stress on the system and the healing process caused by other dysfunctions such as heart disease, diabetes, renal dysfunction);
  - majority of deaths will occur 2-3 weeks post burn, due to sepsis and/or electrolyte imbalance.
— **Primary nursing responsibilities** are to support the aims of treatment which include the prevention and control of (1) shock; (2) electrolyte imbalance; (3) infection; and (4) physical and emotional pain and discomfort.

**Specific Considerations, Potential Patient Outcomes, and Nursing Actions:**

1) Maintenance of Respiratory Function

The patient will have an adequate airway; will be free of complications that result from burn damage to the area or from a compromised respiratory function:
  - know that neck, head & facial burns are early indicators of possible respiratory problems, either from inhalation injury or edema;
  - when edema or other problems exist, pt. may be unable to communicate respiratory difficulties; observe closely for dyspnea, stridor, hoarseness, prolonged expiration & cyanosis; record rate & characteristics of respirations at least Q1H & PRN:
  - know that intubation or a tracheostomy may be utilized as a preventive measure (see NCPG #2:25, "Tracheostomy"); keep emergency tray on hand;
  - turn pt., cough & deep breathe Q2H or as ordered, IPPB may be ordered.

2) Relief of Pain and Discomfort

The patient will maintain a level of comfort that will allow him to accept and/or participate in his care:
  - know that level or amount of pain may not be directly related to burn injury but to systemic attempts to deal with the injury;
  - assessment of level of discomfort should consider depth & extent of injury, areas of involvement, age, other pathology present, & previous treatment;
  - know that if pt. cannot speak or is delirious, the only way s/he may be able to communicate discomfort or pain is through restlessness, abusive behavior, crying, or facial expressions;

— maintain an accurate record of amount, time & type of medication utilized; too much medication, too soon, can cause respiratory difficulties; chart effect on pt.;

— know that sedation or pain medication is generally administered IV to increase adequate absorption; is often given ½ hour prior to debridement procedure & prior to administration of Sulfamylon ointment to ensure pt. comfort & adequate relaxation;

— when necessary to move/turn pt., plan to do so ½ hour after giving pain medication;

— since convalescence will be prolonged, give pain med. cautiously, judiciously & conservatively, ensuring that the pt. is given adequate relief but is not overmedicated;

— refer to NCPG #1:30, "The Patient Experiencing Pain."

**3) Restoration of Fluid and Electrolyte Balance**

The patient will maintain adequate blood volume and fluid and electrolyte balance:

— record weight of pt. on admission or as soon after as possible; measure circumference of burned areas;

— record accurate fluid intake (mouth, IV, etc.) & output (urine, perspiration, etc.) QH; IVs are adjusted according to hourly output; fluid replacement formula most often used is Brooke, which recommends using 1.5 ml. of fluid/kilogram of body surface involved; refer to NCPG #2:46, "IV Therapy";

— assess periodically for signs & symptoms of *inadequate fluid replacement*/impending shock (excessive thirst, restlessness, disorientation, increased pulse, decreased BP, decreased urine output); or of *excessive fluid replacement*/ pulmonary congestion, edema (dyspnea, venous engorgement, moist rales, increased BP, CVP greater than 15 cm. of $H_2O$);

— see NCPGs #3:48 & 49, "Fluids & Electrolytes";

— read lab. results & report those that directly reflect a fluid & electrolyte imbalance to Dr.; most frequent lab. requests include: electrolytes, hemoglobin, hematocrit, serum proteins, serum sodium, BUN & urinalysis;

— when massive tissue damage has occurred, hyperkalemia will result; check with Dr. re: IV orders; give food/fluids low in potassium; see NCPG #2:48, "Potassium Imbalance";

— take vital signs at least Q1H & PRN;

— if CVP line in place, refer to NCPG #2:40, "CVP Line";

— elevate all burned areas possible.

**4) Prevention of Complications**

The patient will be free of complications such as wound infection, pneumonia, shock:

— prepare patient for hydrotherapy; use individual burn unit guidelines for this procedure;

— determine type of isolation techniques to be used; no matter the technique, personnel should wear gowns, gloves & masks to help keep the bacterial count to a minimum;

— know that burn wound sepsis is the most common complication; burn is sterile for first 24 hours; after this period, bacteria contaminate the surface and massively invade the burn wound & surrounding tissue; sepsis usually occurs in full thickness injuries & can result in septicemia & may lead to death; a clean environment, proper handwashing techniques, & use of sterile equipment & supplies are essential to decrease or eliminate transfer of organisms to & from the pt.;

— observe for signs & symptoms of sepsis; earliest is a gradual increase or decrease in temperature; others include leukocytosis, marked increase in respirations & pulse;

— utilize strict sterile technique in changing dressing;

— give antibiotics as ordered, & observe pt. response;

— GI complications (especially Curling's stress ulcers) occur frequently as a response to burn injuries involving a large percent of the body; observe, chart & report to Dr. signs of gastric dilatation, abdominal distention, nausea, vomiting, bleeding, regurgitation, especially in those pts. who may be disoriented.

5) Promotion of Psychosocial Adjustment | The patient will be able to cope with the extent and number of losses and will utilize significant others and situational supports to adapt:

— see NCPG #2:28, "The Burn Patient: Common Behaviors" and NCPG #1:31, "Responses to Loss: The Grief and Mourning Process."

## Discharge Planning and Teaching Objectives/Outcomes

Refer to this section in NCPG #2:06, "The Patient with Burns: Convalescent Phase."

### Recommended References

"Burns: What to do During the First Crucial Hours," by C. Jones and I. Feller. *Nursing '77*, March 1977:22–31.

"Central Venous Pressure Line (CVP). NCP Guide #2:40, 2nd Ed., Nurseco, 1980.

"Emergency Care of Burned Patient," by Mary Wagner. *American Journal of Nursing*, November 1977:1788–1791.

"Fluids and Electrolytes, Parts A & B." NCP Guides #3:48 & 49, Nurseco, 1977.

"Intravenous Therapy: General Principles," NCP Guide #2:46, 2nd Ed., Nurseco, 1980.

"Isolation: Precise Procedure for Better Protection," by Mary Castle. *Nursing '75*, May 1975: 50–58.

"Potassium Imbalance." NCP Guide #2:48, 2nd Ed., Nurseco, 1980.

"Restoring Fluid Balance in Patient with Severe Burns," by P. Rogenes and J. Moylan. *American Journal of Nursing*, December 1976:1952–1957.

"Septic Shock in the Burn Patient." Nursing Grand Rounds. *Nursing '76*, January 1976:38–43.

"Shock, Part II: Different Kinds, Different Problems," by Joy Wiley. *Nursing '74*, May 1974:43–53.

"The Burn Patient: Common Behaviors." NCP Guide #2:28, 2nd Ed., Nurseco, 1980.

"The Patient Experiencing Pain," NCP Guide #1:30, 2nd Ed., Nurseco, 1980.

"The Patient With a Tracheostomy." NCP Guide #2:25, 2nd Ed., Nurseco, 1980.

# The Patient with Burns: Convalescent Phase

**LONG TERM GOAL:**   The patient will achieve maximum physiologic, emotional and functional rehabilitation within the limits of any resultant disability.

**General Considerations:**
— The **primary feature** of the convalescent phase is **care of the burn wound:**
  (1) **Initial care of burn wound:**
    — Aims of treatment are: (a) to remove any eschar, (b) to increase circulation to area, (c) to promote formulation of granulation tissue, and (d) to prepare the wound area for grafting.
    — Commonly-used terms:
    *granulation tissue:* a deep pink, fragile tissue that bleeds easily;
    *eschar:* thick, dry, nonviable tissue which forms over second and third degree burn areas; appears brownish or black;
    *debridement:* removal of eschar at the interface of the living and dead tissue; only dead tissue is removed;
    *escharotomy:* the surgical release of pressure from eschar, resulting in restoration of circulation to the area.
    — Wet soaks are often used to ease the removal of eschar and to reduce edema of granulation tissue.
    — Hydrotherapy is used as a softening method for facilitating debridement of eschar and debris.
  (2) **Methods of wound treatment:**
    — Choice of methods depends on the philosophy of burn team as well as the condition and circumstances of the patient. Major methods include:
      • *Open* (exposure): the burn is exposed to the air to facilitate drying of the exudate and formation of a crust that protects the wound; with this method the environment must be kept free of organisms.
      • *Closed* (pressure dressing): the entire burn surface is covered with a pressure dressing which is changed as soon as exudate appears on the surface.
      • *Topical Antimicrobials:* the wound is covered with ointment, creams or solutions that include an antimicrobial agent; these topical agents are usually covered with a single layer dressing and held in place with a single layer stretch bandage.
      • *Sulfamylon Acetate Ointment:* this specific antimicrobial is used widely because it penetrates the eschar and is relatively nontoxic although it does inhibit carbonic anhydrase activity and may cause metabolic acidosis. *This topical agent causes a burning sensation about ½ hour after administration; therefore administer pain medication prior to each treatment.* When

applied, this agent is put directly over the burned areas with a gloved hand and then covered with a single layer of fine mesh gauze and fastened with a single layer of stretch gauze.
- *Silver Sulfadiazine:* this topical agent is a cream compound of silver and sulfadiazine. It is odorless and there is little pain associated with its application, is particularly effective against both gram-negative and gram-positive microorganisms; is applied over entire wound surface and left exposed, or covered with a single layer of mesh gauze.
- *Silver Nitrate:* not in wide use at this time, although it has been widely used because of its bacteriostatic properties.
- *Garamycin Cream:* the properties are useful against both gram-negative and gram-positive organisms; ointment spreads easily, is not painful but is nephrotoxic, therefore careful monitoring of creatinine levels is necessary; promotes resistant strains which may spread to other patients.
- *Betadine Solution and Providone Iodine Ointment:* can be applied as ointment or sprayed on; is effective against gram-negative and gram-positive organisms, causes some stinging which disappears and causes crust formation.

(3) **Closure of the burn wound:**
— Skin grafts are used to: (a) close an open wound (therefore minimizing chance of infection); (b) prevent fluid loss; and (c) restore appearance and/or function of the affected part. Grafts can be temporary or permanent, and are classed according to source of tissue:
- *Homograft* (allograft): skin graft obtained from living persons or cadavers (used as temporary coverings for extensive burns until person's own skin is ready for grafting); used to decrease loss of water, electrolytes, proteins and body fluids; to reduce pain; to control infection; and to hasten development of granulation tissue.
- *Heterograft* (xenograft): temporary covering of animal skin or synthetic skin; porcine grafts are the ones most widely utilized.
- *Autograft:* graft obtained from an uninjured part of the patient; may be *full-thickness* (those taken at the junction of the dermis and subcutaneous tissue), or *split thickness,* (thin, intermediate or thick, running the gamut of including only part of the dermis to that of inclusion of deeper portions of the dermis); donor sites heal spontaneously.

**Specific Considerations, Potential Patient Outcomes, and Nursing Actions:**

1) Restoration of Skin Integrity — The patient will have wound healing and/or preparation of wound for grafting that is free of site or systemic infection:
— skin-wound cleansing, no matter method of wound treatment, usually involves use of hydrotherapy; assess need for giving pain med. ½ hour prior to cleansing procedure; carry out wound treatment per Dr.'s orders & hospital procedure;
— provide specific care for the pt. receiving skin grafts:
(1) Preoperative:
— maintain an adequate nutritional intake (in order to promote tissue health):

- maintain antibiotic regimen & infection control measures;
- apply wet soaks to injured tissue as ordered;
- identify pt.'s concerns & questions regarding the procedure; provide answers, support & alleviate anxiety re: these concerns;
- see NCPG #2:44, "General Pre-op Care";
(2) Postoperative:
- elevate grafted extremity; prevent injury & movement of affected area;
- avoid excessive pressure on area (due to tight bandages); avoid use of adhesive tape on graft area;
- observe donor site for infection & bleeding;
- use strict aseptic technique in all dressing changes; avoid extremes of temperature in moist dressings;
- see NCPGs #2:41, 42, 43, "General Post-op Care, Parts A, B, C."

**2) Relief of Pain and Discomfort**

The patient will have periods of rest, comfort and freedom from pain;
- see section on Pain in NCPG #2:05, "The Burn Patient: Acute Phase";
- refer to NCPG #1:30, "The Patient Experiencing Pain";
- provide IM pain medication only when ordered or necessary; chance of addiction can be minimized by use of oral pain medication;
- assess pt.'s response to medication; note changes in tolerance & report such changes to Dr.

**3) Prevention of Complications**

The patient will be free of complications including immobility, pressure areas, and infection:
- monitor wound/graft sites for early signs of infection; see section on Complications in NCPG #2:05, "The Burn Patient: Acute Phase";
- when immobilization of a part or area is necessary, provide for proper positioning and/or support of that body part, using soft splints, rolled towels, etc.;
- provide both active & passive range of motion for all body parts; refer to NCPG #1:47, "ROM Exercises";
- give mouth care & eye care to those pts. who are unable to do so themselves; eyes which are open all the time do not lubricate the eyeball & serious eye damage, even loss, can result;
- provide nursing care to prevent hazards of immobility; see NCPG #2:45.

4) Maintenance of Fluid, Electrolyte & Nutritional Balance — The patient will have an adequate intake for cell and tissue growth and development, for body resources to enhance rehabilitation and for activities necessary to meet activities of daily living:
   — administer fluid amts. (both IV & NG tube) strictly as ordered; be alert to signs of fluid & electrolyte imbalance (see NCPGs #3:48 & 49);
   — when using NG tube, ensure that it is properly located in the stomach prior to administration of any fluids or foods;
   — maintain a high protein, high caloric diet; establish frequent small feedings interspersed with, or instead of, usual meals; assess pt. likes & dislikes; work with family & dietician to provide these;
   — provide adequate rest periods for pt. prior to & following meals; ensure that pt. is not too tired to eat;
   — dressing changes should be carried out in advance of meals; this will reduce environmental & physical discomforts associated with the dressing change & odors.

5) Psychosocial Adjustment (to Long Term Treatment & Rehabilitation) — The patient will make the transition from extreme dependence to interdependence on others; will accept the physical assistance necessary for rehabilitation:
   — see NCPG #2:28, "The Burn Patient: Common Behaviors";
   — meet with physical & other rehabilitation therapists to coordinate programs;
   — incorporate pt./family suggestions into planning, implementing & evaluating pt. care;
   — maintain proper positioning & body alignment of pt. at all times (see NCPG #2:45, section on musculoskeletal system).

## Discharge Planning and Teaching Objectives/Outcomes
1) (Patient/Family/Significant Other) Has information about, and has been referred to, community resources to be utilized in the home.
2) Has demonstrated ability to change own dressings safely and adequately.
3) Has appointment with doctor or clinic and a supply of medications to take with him.
4) Has a written plan of daily care including exercises, dietary regimen, medications, dressing changes.
5) Has the telephone number and/or appointment with some person who can act as a resource of support to patient and family upon discharge (ensure the resource person is available and willing).

**Recommended References**
"A Tool for Assessing Families of Burned Children," by L. Tolabere and P. Philips. *American Journal of Nursing*, February 1976:225–227.
"Betsy Was So Little . . . and Her Problems So Big," by Judy Bell. *Nursing '77*, June 1977:34–37.
"The Burn Patient: Common Behaviors." NCP Guide #2:28, 2nd Ed., Nurseco, 1980.
"Commonsense Guide to Topical Burn Therapy," by L. Schumann and S. Gaston. *Nursing '79*, March 1979:34–39.

"Fluids and Electrolytes, Parts A&B." NCP Guides #'s 3:48 & 9, Nurseco, 1977.

"General Pre-op Care." NCP Guide #2:44, 2nd Ed., Nurseco, 1980.

"General Post-op Care." NCP Guides #2:41, 42, 43, 2nd Ed., Nurseco, 1980.

"Hazards of Immobility." NCP Guide #2:45, 2nd Ed., Nurseco, 1980.

"Individual Burn Wound Dressings," by Florence Jacoby. *Nursing '77*, June 1977:62–68.

"The Patient Experiencing Pain." NCP Guide #1:30, 2nd Ed., Nurseco, 1980.

"The Patient With Burns: Critical-Acute Phase." NCP Guide #2:05, 2nd Ed., Nurseco, 1980.

"Porcine Skin Dressings for Burns," by Velda Stinson. *American Journal of Nursing*, January 1974:111–112.

"Range of Motion Exercises." NCP Guide #1:47, 2nd Ed., Nurseco, 1980.

"Responses to Loss: the Grief and Mourning Process." NCP Guide #1:31, 2nd Ed., Nurseco, 1980.

"Surgery of Burns." *Surgical Clinics of North America*, Philadelphia, W.B. Saunders Co., December 1970.

# The Patient with Diabetes

**Definition:** Diabetes mellitus is a chronic, metabolic disorder which affects the body's ability to manufacture and/or utilize insulin (the hormone produced by the beta cells of the pancreas).

**LONG TERM GOAL:** The patient will reach and maintain the optimum level of performance possible, living within the limits of the disease and treatment regimen, preventing as much as possible the pathological changes and complications of diabetes; the patient will accept and integrate successfully the diabetic lifestyle into self-concept and will achieve self-confident control; the patient will resume normal home, family, community roles with necessary adaptation.

## General Considerations:
— **Incidence:** directly affects 10 million Americans (over 50 million affected indirectly via family ties); incidence increasing yearly; probability increases with age and obesity; disease found more commonly in women, in non-whites, in those with yearly incomes of under $5000.
— **Types: Juvenile**—onset before 39 years of age, usually insulin-dependent, a virus has been implicated as a possible causal factor; **Mature**—onset in later years, often controlled by diet alone or with oral med., causal factors related to obesity and heredity. **Diagnosis** includes a fasting blood sugar, 2 Hr. Post-Prandial, and a thorough physical & history.
— **Signs and Symptoms:** Frequent urination (polyuria), excessive thirst (polydipsia), fatigue, loss of weight associated with excessive hunger (polyphagia), and chronic infections slow to heal. Peripheral neuropathy (diminished sensations) is common.
— **Treatment** aims: to control symptoms and to prevent or control complications associated with metabolic, neurologic, and cardiovascular consequences of the disease. **Education** of the patient and family is the keystone of quality care, whether the patient is newly diagnosed, or is a re-admission for surgery, illness, injury or associated complication.
— **Nursing responsibilities** (whether hospital staff, metabolic clinic, home health or occupational RN) involve assessment, education, counseling and assisting the patient and family to accept and cope effectively in the long-term management of this lifetime condition. After consulting with the physician re: the therapeutic regimen or prescribed diet, drugs, exercise and follow-up care, the nurse should interview the patient and family to determine what they know, what they need to know, and what their expectations are regarding hospitalization, treatment and care after discharge. In collaboration with them, establish objectives and plans for what should be taught, when and by whom. Obtain and review educational materials for them, which will be relevant and useful. Suggested teaching outcomes are given below.

## Specific Considerations, Potential Patient Outcomes, and Nursing Actions:
1) Nutrition        The patient establishes and maintains ideal body weight and proper nutrition; the patient eats all food at proper times and does not eat between meal snacks, except as prescribed; the patient is able to meet dietary requirements in a liquid form whenever s/he is unable to chew, take solid foods, has missed or failed to finish a complete meal:

— give all meals & snacks on time; encourage full consumption; record & measure amounts left & give replacement carbohydrate feeding;

— administer vitamin & mineral supplements as ordered;

— see NCPG #1:36, "General Dietary Principles for the Diabetic," & NCPG #1:37, "Liquid Diet Substitutes for the Diabetic"; teach pt. & family about dietary planning or refer to teaching dietician for this.

**2) Medications**   The patient receives insulin or oral hypoglycemics as ordered; the patient knows about the different types of insulin, how to store and prepare for an injection; how to give own injections correctly, rotating sites according to a plan, and how to care for equipment safely:

— see NCPG #1:38, "Properties of Insulin Preparations"; teach pt. & family about insulin, its storage & handling, activity & effects;

— teach pt. & at least one family member to administer insulin correctly, safely & satisfactorily;

— teach pt. & family the factors that increase insulin need (trauma, infection, fever, exposure to cold, the adrenal hormones-catecholamines increased by stress & tension) & to avoid these factors when possible; if these influences are unavoidable, then to seek prompt medical advice;

— teach the importance & method of site rotation & provide a suitable chart for recording sites used with dates.

**3) Exercise**   The patient maintains a normal activity level for age to provide a balance for insulin and diet being given; the patient demonstrates the knowledge that exercise is an important part of treatment by being physically active on a daily basis:

— teach pt. that regular physical exercise done at least three times a week for 20 min. each time has the following benefits: *decreases* BP, body weight, appetite, tension, triglycerides and need for some insulin; (exercise) *increases* stamina, self-confidence and work performance;

— teach pt. to prepare for exercise by adjusting medication & food; have pt. be prepared (carry on person) with some form of quick acting sugar (jelly beans, Life Savers, Cake Mate Decorating Jell) in case of need;

— see recommended references for book on sports & exercise.

**4) Prevention of Complications**   The patient knows the common complications of diabetes (arteriosclerosis, chronic infections, eye trouble, neuritis, heart disease, kidney disease) and most of the early warning signs to report to his doctor; the patient and family can describe the difference between insulin reaction and ketoacidosis, can tell what to do for each situation; the patient and family demonstrate knowledge of good oral hygiene, proper skin and foot care and what to do for illness:

— know that the *first step* to preventing complications is *assessment* of the possibilities and recognition of the importance of the pt. having informed, self-confident control of his disease;

— hold frequent *conferences* with physician, dietician, social worker & other staff members to discuss pt.'s progress, to exchange suggestions & observations, to coordinate the treatment plan & teaching;

— *teach pt.* & *family* about *ketoacidosis* & *hypoglycemia*; refer to NCPG #1:35;

— evaluate pt.'s foot care needs; demonstrate proper *foot care* & supervise return demonstrations; see NCPG #1:39:

— know that glucose in the epidermis of diabetic pts. predisposes to *skin infections*; observe & report skin lesions; prevent chafing & irritation caused by perspiration by powdering skin surfaces & by teaching pt. to wear loose-fitting cotton garments next to skin;

— observe & report lesions of mouth, *gum and teeth conditions*; teach & supervise proper dental hygiene (including use of dental floss & disclosing tablets); refer to dentist PRN & follow-up to ensure this is done;

— know that blurred vision can result from changed glucose levels and insulin dosages: cataracts, glaucoma & retinopathy are also common; refer for *opthalmology evaluation* after condition stabilizes for two months & thereafter on a regular basis as recommended by progress of disease;

— check pt.'s *weight and BP* regularly; assess for weight gain, edema, gradual hypertension, anginal pains & report accordingly;

— assess for *peripheral vascular disease*; check pedal pulses, ulcerations & infections of feet & legs; note presence of intermittent claudication (leg pain only while walking);

— assess for *peripheral neuropathy*; note impaired sensation of feet & fingers; teach pt. caution while cooking, lighting matches, smoking, using heating appliances, being around extreme sources of heat or cold;

— observe & check for itching or burning on *urination*, diminished output, increased specific gravity, flank pain, urgency, frequency, dysuria, pneumaturia (bubbly voided urine due to action of bacteria upon glucose in urine); record & report all abnormal signs & symptoms; teach pt. & family to do this after discharge;

— remind pt. never to take patent or non-prescribed medicines (which may contain high amts. of sugar in flavoring or additives) unless their doctor knows & gives approval;

— teach pt. & family what to do in case of *minor short-term illness* (cold or flu, etc.):

    (1) *take insulin* as regularly prescribed (or regularly prescribed oral hypoglycemics, if tolerated) unless & until s/he can reach doctor;

    (2) go to bed & keep warm;

    (3) take fluids as tolerated every hour & keep a record of what taken & how much;

    (4) if s/he can't take solid foods, replace usual diet with semi-liquid carbohydrates (same number of grams); refer to NCPG #1:37, "Liquid Diet Substitutes for the Diabetic";

(5) test urine for sugar & acetone *at least* every four hours & keep a record of results;

(6) be in touch with doctor by phone, so s/he can monitor progress; if illness lasts more than 48 hours, or if symptoms grow worse, *see* doctor; notify doctor immediately for vomiting or diarrhea, because they upset the fluid & electrolyte balance quickly & reduce the blood sugar & insulin requirements; *remember* infection, fever & stress increase the need for insulin even if pt. can't eat normally, so insulin must be taken when ill;

— provide pt. with ID card for wallet indicating: doctor's name & address, types of medication being taken & how much, next of kin to be notified in emergency, & other pertinent information; an ID bracelet is more visible & quickly noticed, so help pt. arrange for getting one;

— urge pt. to visit doctor or clinic at least two months prior to taking an extended trip (especially outside country), so that minor health problems can be detected & corrected, so that immunization reactions have completed their course, so that adequate plans & precautions are considered; see recommended references for additional info; have pt. assemble all diabetic supplies & doctor's statement in "carry-on" hand luggage; tell pt. s/he can obtain additional info from: The International Diabetes Foundation, 3-6 Alfred Place, London, WCIE, 7EE, England.

5) Urine Testing    The patient will assess control daily by testing urine correctly and keeping records; the patient and at least one family member or friend will demonstrate the two-drop Clinitest method and the Acetest:

— teach pt. an appropriate method of testing urine after considering pt. needs & medications, advantages & disadvantages of products, & physician preference; refer to NCPG #1:50, "Teaching Patients—Skills and Procedures";

— explain reasons for not touching tablets or testing paper with fingers;

— know that medications & vitamins may affect results (ex. Vit. C & levodopa cause false negatives with Tes-Tape; Keflin, Aspirin & Vit. C cause false positives with Clinitests) so if pt. is taking drugs other than insulin, discuss appropriate testing material with pharmacist & physician;

— although research results are controversial, know that it is probably best to use a second, freshly voided specimen following a previous emptying of bladder; teach pt. reasons for doing so;

— know that percentage of sugar has differing "plus" meanings on various products so *record results in percentages only* & name the test used; teach the pt. & other staff to do so, as consistency is essential for correctly & effectively regulating insulin dosage; provide record form for listing results (including one for taking home);

— know that if pt. has over 2% sugar (a bright orange "pass through" phenomenon, when glycosuria is too high to react accurately), you should use & teach pt. the *"2 drop test"* (2 drops urine with 10 drops water) to further determine correct percentage of sugar, but you must *use a different color chart*;

— for visually impaired pts., teach the "touch test" (add baking soda to urine in a test tube, cover with a finger cot, feel the inflation caused by gaseous expansion showing presence of sugar) or use Mega-Diastix;

— for nursing mothers and pregnant women in third trimester, use an enzyme test (Tes-Tape, Diastix) to check for *glyco*suria because Clinitest will be positive for *lactose* in urine;

— for older persons, know that renal threshold for glucose rises with age, so pt. may be hyperglycemic without glycosuria, therefore, postprandial blood sugars may be needed.

6) Psychosocial Adjustment

The patient will demonstrate a productive, self-reliant adjustment to diabetic condition and management; the patient (and family) will express feelings of acceptance, self-confidence and relief of fear concerning condition:

— see NCPG #1:44, "Suggestions for Interviewing"; consult both pt. & family for assistance in planning, implementing & evaluating teaching program; refer to NCPG #1:49, "Teaching Patients: General Suggestions";

— observe family relationships to estimate degree of support available to pt. after discharge; consider enlisting the aid of a close friend PRN;

— provide pt. & family with address & phone number of local diabetes assn; encourage them to attend monthly lecture series & to participate in self-help groups; give them pamphlets to take home for future reference;

— know & be informed about diabetes-related sexual & reproductive malfunctions which may occur & which doubtlessly concern pt.; see recommended references; provide sound explanations with sympathetic counseling to alleviate anxiety associated with problem;

— know that emotional upsets & tension increase need for insulin; attempt to determine & alleviate causes of stress or help pt. to cope more effectively; provide opportunities for pt./family to express feelings, concerns, frustrations & annoyances;

— assess need for convalescent hospital or home health care assistance & make appropriate referrals.

## Discharge Planning and Teaching Objectives/Outcomes

1) (Patient/Family/Significant Other) Can answer questions: What is diabetes, what are the common symptoms, treatment and expectations for its control? Has received at least one current pamphlet on diabetes and a written sheet of instructions regarding special aspects of condition.

2) Can test urine properly for sugar and acetone; knows how to keep an accurate record.

3) Can tell about types of insulin, how to store and handle it correctly; can give own injections accurately and safely, rotating sites according to a plan and caring for equipment without contamination.

4) Can state the differing symptoms and signs of hypoglycemia and ketoacidosis; knows exactly what to do for each situation.

5) Maintains a blood glucose of 80-200 mg.%; maintains a negative urine and acetone level.

6) Has a printed sheet of dietary instructions and sample menus. Can understand, accept and help plan a well-balanced meal consistent with prescribed grams of protein, carbohydrate, fat and calories needed to maintain ideal weight. Knows the general dietary rules of food measurement and preparation. Can list the foods allowed and those to avoid.

7) Can describe the meaning and importance of good personal health habits, including regular, moderate exercise; daily care of teeth, skin and feet; adequate rest and sleep; regular medical check-ups (including opthamologist and dentist).

8) Knows the common complications of diabetes (arteriosclerosis, chronic infections, eye trouble, skin lesions, neuritis, heart disease, kidney ailments) and the early warning signs to report to a doctor.

9) Has an identification card in wallet, which includes the name, address and phone number of next of kin, of physician, of self, as well as the names and dosages of medications, and what to do for an insulin reaction.

10) Knows the name and address of the American Diabetes Association and its local chapter. Is aware of the services available and knows of the availability of community health services in the home if necessary or desirable.

**Recommended References**

"Better Use of Resources Equals Better Health for Diabetics," by June Isaf and Maria Alogna. *American Journal of Nursing*, November 1977:1792–1795.

"Deliver Facts To Help Diabetics Plan Parenthood," by Catherine Garofano. *Nursing 77*, April 1977:13–16.

*Diabetes Care, Diabetes Forecast*, and other current literature. American Diabetes Association, 600 Fifth Ave., New York, NY 10020.

"Diagnosis and Management of Diabetes in the Elderly," by Charlotte Eliopoulos. *American Journal of Nursing*, May 1978:884–887.

"Differentiating Hypoglycemia and Ketoacidosis," *NCP Guide* #1:35, 2nd. Ed., Nurseco, 1980.

*Education and Management of the Patient with Diabetes*. Ames Co., Div. Miles Laboratories, Inc., P O Box 70, Elkhart, IN 46515.

"General Dietary Principles for the Diabetic," *NCP Guide* #1:36, 2nd. Ed., Nurseco, 1980.

"Liquid Diet Substitutes for the Diabetic," *NCP Guide* #1:37, 2nd. Ed., Nurseco, 1980.

*Managing Diabetics Properly*. Nursing 78 Books, Intermed Communications, Inc., Horsham, PA 19044.

*Managing Your Diabetes*, by Jean Ranch and Mae McWeeny. Abbot-Northwestern Hospital, Inc., 1978. (from Minneapolis Med. Center Publications Office, 810 E. 27th St., Minn., MN 55407).

"Properties of Insulin Preparations," *NCP Guide* #1:38, 2nd. Ed., Nurseco, 1980.

"Recommended Care of the Feet for Diabetics," *NCP Guide* #1:39, 2nd. Ed., Nurseco, 1980.

"Reporting Urine Test Results: Switch from + to %," by Dorothy Lundin. *American Journal of Nursing*, May 1978:878,879.

"Suggestions for Interviewing," *NCP Guide* #1:44, 2nd. Ed., Nurseco, 1980.

"Teaching Patients: General Suggestions," *NCP Guide* #1:49, 2nd. Ed., Nurseco, 1980.

"Teaching Patients: Specific Plan for Skills and Procedures," *NCP Guide* #1:50, 2nd. Ed., Nurseco, 1980.

*The Diabetics Sports and Exercise Book*, by J. Biermann and B. Toohey. J.B. Lippincott Co., Philadelphia, 1977.

"Travel Tips for the Peripatetic Diabetic," by Catherine Garofano. *Nursing 77*, August 1977:44–46.

"When a Pregnant Woman Is Diabetic." *American Journal of Nursing*, March 1979:448–458.

# The Patient with Emphysema, Pulmonary

**Definition:** An irreversible condition in which there is dilatation of all the finer air passages, plus dilatation and coalesence of the alveoli resulting in loss of elasticity, trapping of air, and chronic hyperextension of the lungs.

**LONG TERM GOAL:** The patient will carry out activities of daily living within limitations and regimen imposed by the medical diagnosis, and will learn preventive measures designed to retard progress of the disease.

## General Considerations:

— Pulmonary emphysema is one of three conditions collectively known as chronic, obstructive pulmonary disease (COPD); the other two are chronic bronchitis and asthma. Frequently, patients suffer from elements of all three.

— It usually **occurs** as the end result of chronic bronchial irritation and infection, which leads to edema, mucus production, bronchospasm, constriction of the finer airways, and loss of lung elasticity. It occurs most often in persons over 45 years of age who have a long history of cigarette smoking.

— There is no cure for the disease but its progress can be arrested in great part by maintenance of good, general health, avoidance of smoking, and control of air pollution.

— **Nursing responsibilities** include carrying out measures to resolve the acute conditions and teaching the patient/family/significant other preventive measures which will arrest progress of the disease and maintain optional pulmonary function.

## Specific Considerations, Potential Patient Outcomes, and Nursing Actions:

1) Respiratory Dysfunction     The patient will maintain a patent airway; will breathe with as little effort as possible; will expectorate mucus:

— place pt. in an upright position, supporting back & arms (with pillow on over-bed table);

— check with Dr. re: giving $O_2$; the usual amt. is 1-2 liters/min., *no more* than 3 (otherwise, pt. may retain $CO_2$ which could lead to respiratory arrest); if $O_2$ given, administer it *continuously*, not intermittently;

— instruct pt. to use pursed-lip breathing during episodes of dypsnea;

— know that these pts. produce large amts. of thick sputum that is difficult to expectorate; suction PRN;

— provide adequate hydration (to liquefy secretions); check with Dr. re: fluid restrictions (related to existing cardiac or fluid problems); with no restrictions, ensure an intake of at least 2000cc's daily;

— provide humidification with warm steam or as Dr. orders, to aid expectoration;

— work with respiratory therapist re: scheduling of treatments & follow-up measures; with no respiratory therapist available, collaborate with Dr. re: postural drainage, IPPB & percussion/vibration to lower lobes;

— explain to pt. how the acute conditions (infection, respiratory failure/acidosis or whatever they are) impact upon his breathing & the expected results of treatment; be aware that acute SOB is a very frightening experience for the pt. & that giving information is an effective way to decrease fear & anxiety.

— observe for early signs of $CO_2$ narcosis (confusion, lethargy, deep sleep, changes in respiratory rate or depth, inability to help with own care) & report to Dr. at once; DC $O_2$.

**2) Control of Infection**

The patient will achieve resolution of acute episode; will be free of preventable infections:

— give antibiotics on time to maintain a constant level in blood;

— place pt. in a private room if possible, or at least away from any pt. with an infection;

— know that these pts. are especially susceptible to infections due to their chronic, debilitated condition;

— prevent staff & visitors with colds or other infections from going into pt.'s room;

— keep a large supply of tissues at bedside within easy reach of pt.;

— ensure that room is damp-dusted in an effort to cut down air pollution;

— check environmental controls: avoid draughts, chilling, extreme temperatures.

**3) Energy Conservation**

The patient will spread out energy demands over the day; the patient will avoid becoming extremely fatigued:

— know that these pts. have a limited amt. of energy, that energy is one of their most precious commodities, & that much of it is consumed with eating & talking;

— be aware that these pts. will have less energy in early am. due to accumulation of secretions during the night; postpone am. activities until they have expectorated the mucus;

— help pt. discover own point of fatigue, & to not go beyond that;

— ensure that pt. knows & carries out breathing exercises on a daily basis, & knows how to do pursed-lip breathing;

— keep pt.'s supplies close at hand so that s/he can reach them easily;

— schedule adequate rest periods between treatments, meals, tests, visitors, etc. to prevent pt. from becoming fatigued.

**4) Patient Teaching Program**

The patient will be able to do postural drainage, breathing exercises; will develop a plan to conserve energy:

— assess pt.'s ability to carry out postural drainage, percussion & vibration; collaborate with respiratory therapist to teach these procedures PRN;

— check pt.'s status re: breathing exercises; if pt. needs to strengthen muscles of expiration, suggest this:

a) Do for 10-15 mins. TID: Patient in recumbent position, with one hand on abdomen and other on upper chest; inhale through nose, raising abdomen against hand; exhale while pursing lips, contracting the abdominal muscles, and moving abdomen inward; chest should not move. As patient can tolerate it, sand bags may be added to increase intra-abdominal pressure.

    b) Do for 10 mins. TID: Take a full deep breath. Exhale slowly with pursed lips, blowing out a candle flame, but not extinguishing it. Flame should be 6" away; gradually increase 2"/day to a distance of 36".

— as the acute condition resolves, ensure that pt. takes an active part in his care; allowing him to "just sit" & not participate may literally be deadly for him; his life depends upon learning to provide himself with an adequate pulmonary toilet;

— discuss with pt. his needs for rest, exercise, activity & help him adjust his energy resources accordingly;

— discuss the impact of air pollution, smoking, infections on his body; teach the action & possible side effects of his medications; teach signs of an impending problem or URI (chest tightness, change in color or amt. of sputum, chest pain, excessive fatigue); discuss the role of adequate nutrition & prevention of infection.

## Discharge Planning and Teaching Objectives/Outcomes

1) (Patient/Family/Significant Other) Accepts diagnosis and recognizes that life can be useful, satisfying and worthwhile; knows that pulmonary function can be improved and maintained by adherence to prescribed regimen.

2) Verbalizes knowledge of the purpose and demonstrates satisfactorily postural drainage, aerosol therapy, breathing exercises, and room humidifiers.

3) States the actions and possible side effects of medication s/he is taking; has a supply of medicines to take home and knows where and when to obtain refills.

4) Identifies adequate knowledge of signs and symptoms of impending infection or other problems and knows to contact Dr./clinic at once.

5) Gives evidence of planning to maintain good health habits (adequate food and fluid intake, realistic level of rest and exercise, prevention of infection, avoidance of crowds, smoke-filled rooms, and air pollution.)

### Recommended References
"Acute Respiratory Insufficiency," by Hannelore Sweetwood, RN, BS. *Nursing '77*, December 1977:24–31.

"Better Ways to Cope With C.O.P.D.," by Margaret F. Fuhr, RN, MSN and Alice M. Stein, RN, MA. *Nursing '76*, February 1976:28–38.

*Fall-Winter Advice for Patients With Respiratory Problems*. Respicare Service of Union Carbide Corp., 3 Westchester Plaza, Elmsford, NY 10523.

"Teaching Patients: General Suggestions," *NCP Guide* #1:49, 2nd Ed., Nurseco, 1980.

"Teaching Patients: Specific Plan for Skills and Procedures," *NCP Guide* #1:50, 2nd Ed., Nurseco, 1980.

# The Patient with a Hemorrhoidectomy

**Definition:** Hemorrhoidectomy is a surgical ligation and excision of the dilated blood vessels in the anal region, external to the sphincter and, if needed, submucosal vessels above the internal sphincter.

**LONG TERM GOAL:** The patient will recover from a hemorrhoidectomy free of complications; the patient will return to usual roles in home/job/community after a normal short convalescence.

## General Considerations:

— **Medical treatment** for small hemorrhoids that are mild and uncomplicated consists of a low roughage diet, increased exercise for those with sedentary lifestyles, sitz baths for relief of pain and itching, anesthetic ointments, stool softeners and lubricant suppositories.

— Fear of surgery and pain cause many persons to refuse surgery for as long as possible, even after several episodes of severe pain, bleeding, prolapse and near strangulation. Nurses can help people to reduce their anxiety and to accept an operation when it is recommended.

— **Preop nursing care responsibilities** include operative and anesthetic consents, a perianal prep, tap water enemas until clear, liquid low residue diet, pre-anesthetic medications, voiding or foley catheter placement and oft needed reassurance and explanations.

## Specific Postop Considerations, Potential Patient Outcomes and Nursing Actions:

1) Rest and Comfort

The patient will experience prompt, effective relief of pain as needed; the patient will experience reduced tension, embarrassment, aggression and other nonproductive behaviors associated with severe anal discomfort:

— give narcotics & sedatives as frequently as ordered; don't wait for pt. requests which may be delayed for one reason or another;

— keep fresh ice packs over anal dressing until packing is removed; then astringent, tepid, moist compresses may be ordered;

— anesthetic/antibiotic ointments may be ordered, although excessive use may delay wound healing;

— position pt. on abdomen or side with pillow supports;

— change dressings, T-binders, bedding to keep area clean, dry, comfortable;

— have pt. take 15-20 min. warm sitz baths QID & PRN; have a foam ring or towel in tub for sitting comfort; observe for dizziness, oversedation or weakness & do not leave pt. alone;

— show sympathetic, sensitive, yet tactful concern; avoid embarrassing remarks or questionable humor.

| 2) Prevention of Complications | The patient will have bleeding and infection prevented or promptly controlled: |
|---|---|

— monitor & record TPR and B/P noting quality & changes;
— note restlessness, anxiety, weakness or other behavior change;
— observe for continuing, bright red bleeding & passage of clots; report this to doctor, put pt. to bed, apply ice bag over an absorbent pressure dressing & watch closely.

**3) Nutrition** The patient will resume a regular diet as tolerated after initially taking a liquid to soft low residue diet:
— give liquid to soft low residue diet to postpone first defecation until some healing has taken place & there is less chance of bleeding or infection;
— after recording the first bowel movement, a regular diet is given.

**4) Voiding** The patient will resume normal urinary output without bladder distention:
— urge & record oral fluids, especially tea & coffee if permitted;
— palpate supra-pubic region for distention or ascertain that catheter (if placed) is unkinked & continually patent;
— measure each voided amt. separately to assess retention;
— help male pts. stand to void; help females into sitting position on bedside commode; rinse perineum & change anal dressing after voiding;
— try sitz baths (or Urecholine type injections if ordered) to stimulate voiding & avoid catheterization except as a last resort.

**5) Defecation** The patient will achieve satisfactory bowel movements with as little strain and pain as possible:
— administer laxatives & low retention enema when ordered;
— have pt. take a sitz bath prior to defecation attempt in order to relax & to facilitate removal of cellulose gauze spool used for hemostasis;
— administer narcotic injection for pain relief at least 20-30 min. prior to elimination effort;
— help pt. to bathroom, provide privacy, but remain close by in case of dizziness or other need;
— after defecation, have pt. rest for a few minutes, then take a short sitz bath to cleanse peri-anal region & to promote healing & comfort.

## Discharge Planning and Teaching Objectives/Outcomes

1) (Patient/Family/Significant Other) Has written appointment, date and time for follow-up visit to surgeon.
2) Has obtained (or knows how to get) a foam ring or cushion for sitting comfort.
3) States s/he knows about diet, laxatives, pain medications, sitz baths, safety precautions, need for exercise and expectations for being permitted to drive a car, sit for long periods, return to work, etc.

# The Patient with Hepatitis

**Definition:** Hepatitis is an inflammation and injury of the liver caused by chemical substances (toxic hepatitis), different viruses or other organisms, e.g. gonococcus, streptococcus (viral hepatitis).

**LONG TERM GOAL:** The patient will accept illness and recover to the point that s/he is willing and able to complete convalescence at home with medical guidance; the patient will return to normal roles in home/job/community.

## General Considerations:
— **Signs and Symptoms:** dark urine, clay-colored stools, yellow sclera, jaundice, N&V, anorexia, fatigue, malaise, myalgia, headache, fever; may also have cough, pharyngitis, photophobia; rash, hives, edema and pruritis also possible.
— Viral hepatitis is most commonly of two types: serum hepatitis (type B) or infectious hepatitis (type A). **Both** may be transmitted orally (food, water, fingers contaminated by urine, feces, saliva, semen) or parenterally (blood or blood product-contaminated syringes, needles, dental & surgical instruments, ear piercing tools, etc.) A new Type C Hepatitis has been found in patients who have had multiple transfusions.
— **Incubation period:** 2-4 mos. for SH and 2-8 wks. for IH; exceptions have been recorded.
— **Treatment** to heal and regenerate the liver depends upon adequate rest (often in bed, 2 weeks to 2 months) and a balanced, nutritious, high carbohydrate-low fat diet. Regularly repeated liver function blood studies (SGOT, SGPT, alkaline phosphatase, serum bilirubin, iceterus index, pro time) indicate the effectiveness of treatment and progress of recovery (4-24 weeks).
— **Nursing responsibilities** include health teaching, isolation precautions and procedures designed to minimize outbreaks (e.g. careful handling of bodily secretions, blood and blood products, needles and syringes; no eating policies in hemodialysis, oncology, hematology or blood-donor units; proper housekeeping practices and thorough hand washing habits before and after patient care).

## Specific Considerations, Potential Patient Outcomes, and Nursing Actions:
1) Rest and Comfort
The patient's liver cells will heal and regenerate with minimal residual liver damage:
— bed rest for one or more weeks with use of private bath & toilet facilities is common, if pt. was previously healthy;
— passive & active range-of-motion exercises should be taught & done twice daily; refer to NCPG #1:47;
— provide stress-reducing activities that will encourage rest & relaxation; arrange for sensory stimulation (TV, radio, books, clock, calendar, pictures, hobbies, etc.) & social contacts (visits by friends, family & available staff);
— query pt. re: medications being taken; those which are metabolized in the liver (birth control pills, Dilantin, sedatives, tranquilizers, others) are to be avoided during the acute illness period;
— provide regular skin care, using baths & lotions for dry, itching skin; use decubitus & pressure prevention measures.

2) Nutrition
The patient maintains an optimum fluid, electrolyte, nutritional balance refraining from foods and liquids harmful to the liver:
— administer parenteral fluids with vitamin & mineral supplements as prescribed during the acute phase, especially when the

pt. is anorexic, or has nausea & vomiting;
— when tolerated, serve Hi Pro-Hi CHO-Lo Fat diet in six, small feedings daily; arrange for someone to be present so pt. does not have to eat alone; consult dietician for cultural preferences or special needs;
— hard candy to increase carbohydrate level is no longer advised because it further depresses the appetite for nutritious foods; instead, fresh or canned fruits & juices are provided & encouraged;
— alcohol must be avoided for 4-6 mos. to prevent relapse or prolong convalescence; peanuts, chocolate, ice cream and other fatty foods & snacks are to be avoided as well.

3) Isolation Precautions

The spread of the hepatitis virus will be contained and cross-contamination will be prevented:
— wear gowns, but caps & masks are usually not necessary; gloves are recommended for handling all body secretions;
— tissues, toothbrushes, bed linens, other patient care items require special handling according to hospital procedure;
— carefully dispose of all disposable needles, syringes, IV equipment, paper food service items;
— teach pt. & family necessary precautions, indicating which will be continued after the pt. goes home; kissing is not permitted; the pt. must not prepare or handle food for others; a private bathroom should be provided or care taken to keep the basin and toilet scrupulously clean;
— hand washing is a must for staff, visitors & pt.; a mask should be worn by the pt. if s/he is prone to coughing, sneezing;
— reassure pt. that precautions are temporary; pt. should not be rejected, left alone for long periods or neglected.

4) Prevention of Complications

The patient will be free of preventable complications or have them promptly recognized and managed:
— observe & record changes in pt.'s physical or mental status; note signs of disorientation, irritability, depression; look for ascites, edema, asterixis (metabolic tremor);
— note new bruises or petechiae; observe bleeding from needle sites;
— record color of urine & stools, observing for presence of bleeding, & signs of shock that come with blood loss.

## Discharge Planning and Teaching Objectives/Outcomes

1) (Patient/Family/Significant Other) Understands status of own hepatitis and expresses willingness to adhere to treatment.
2) Has a written list of foods permitted and disallowed on diet; can state a typical day's menu; indicates an appreciation of need to eat at least every three hours to spare liver from unnecessary metabolic work.
3) Has been assisted to complete job disability insurance forms and to make home care arrangements according to need. Knows s/he must not return to any strenuous work or fatiguing activities until doctor has given permission.

**Recommended References**
"Range of Motion Exercises," *NCP Guide* #1:47, 2nd Ed., Nurseco, 1980.
"Viral Hepatitis," by Karen Baranowski, Harry Green II, and J. Thomas Lamont. *Nursing 76*, May 1976:31-38.

# The Patient with Hypertension

**Definition:** Hypertension, according to the American Heart Association, is simply an unstable or persistent elevation of blood pressure above the normal range.

**LONG TERM GOAL:** The patient will reach an optimum level of functioning within a therapeutic program and a modified lifestyle necessary to control his blood pressure throughout his life.

**General Considerations:**

— Persons with a consistent **systolic BP reading equal to or greater than 160 mm. Hg.** and a **diastolic reading greater than 90 mm. Hg.,** generally are considered to be hypertensive and in need of medical evaluation.

— **Incidence:** Estimated at one adult in six in US; more prevalent in women, in black people, often those between 30 & 50 years of age, and in obese persons. Most hypertensives are undiagnosed because of a lack of symptoms ("the hidden disease"); of those who are known, most have "primary" or "essential" type.

— **Causes & Types:** Kidney disease, an adrenal tumor, toxemia of pregnancy and birth control pills are sometimes causes of high blood pressure. In the absence of a known cause, hypertension is typed *essential* or *primary*. It may also be classified as *benign* (slow onset, minimal symptoms) or *malignant* (degenerated and occluded peripheral blood vessels).

— **Treatment aims:** To reduce arterial pressure, to arrest atherosclerosis and to curtail progressive arteriolar disease. To maintain the blood pressure within safe levels, a patient must faithfully adhere to a program of diet, drugs, balanced rest/relaxation/exercise/work schedule and periodic medical check-ups.

— **Low compliance** is a major (& common, 3 out of 4) problem among hypertensives. Reasons given by patients for discontinuing treatment regimen include: felt well, couldn't afford medications, had disagreeable side effects from prescribed drugs, feared dependency on drugs, felt embarrassed or guilty about need to take medicine daily even when symptom-free, received poor or inadequate instruction from medical personnel, took conflicting advice of friends, and/or became discouraged or dissatisfied with continuing treatment, long waits and seeing different doctors during clinic visits, and depersonalization attitude of professional staff.

— **Nursing responsibilities:** Case-finding efforts to detect the unknown, untreated hypertensive; assessment of patient & family for planning, implementing and evaluating a simple, satisfying and successful treatment regimen; and effective education to ensure life-long compliance. Close cooperation between nursing colleagues in the out-patient and in-patient settings (including community health staff) is important to obtain cooperation of patient and a consistent, congruent approach to patient/family.

— The **patient must "own" his disease**, assume responsibility for own health, but must be made to feel that someone cares whether s/he does or not. Support should come from loving family members, concerned significant others and empathetic health care providers. If s/he is to avoid repeated hospitalizations and a worsening illness (serious complications are myocardial infarction, congestive heart failure, stroke and progressive renal failure), s/he must **accept** lifelong hypertensive condition requiring medication to control it even when s/he doesn't feel bad.

## Specific Considerations, Potential Patient Outcomes, and Nursing Actions:

1) Nutrition

The patient will accept and adhere to a low sodium, weight control diet to eliminate overweight, to prevent edema, to reduce the work load of the heart and to lower the blood pressure to satisfactory levels:

— assess pt. attitudes toward food, cooking, seasonings & meal times, so as to gauge motivation to learn & to plan more effective teaching;

— estimate the probable effect that altered food preparation will have on family; learn the family's attitude, beliefs about the pt.'s need for special diet & the degree of willingness to cooperate;

— teach pt./family that sodium restriction will reduce blood volume, thereby lessening the work of the heart;

— confer with dietician re: pt.'s likes & dislikes, cultural preferences, special needs, in order to plan an acceptable diet while in the hospital & to teach effectively about the diet recommended after discharge;

— help the pt. to understand & accept a low sodium weight control diet;

— record daily weight & I & O; note foods left on tray & discuss reason;

— teach pt. what food seasonings do not contain sodium & what salt substitutes are permissible & safe to use; teach pt. to check food labels carefully for sodium compounds;

— teach pt. that caffeine is a vasoconstrictor which increases heart's work & that coffee, tea, cola drinks & chocolate have caffeine;

— refer to NCPG #3:44, "Low Sodium Diets";

— give pt./family written dietary instructions to read & keep.

2) Rest and Exercise

The patient will experience reduced physical and emotional tension; the patient's circulation and muscle tone will be improved; the patient will explore new ways of coping more effectively with stress:

— recommend & provide for daily walks, up to 30 min. depending on physical status & activity tolerance;

— encourage the pt. to decide to participate more actively in some sport (golf, tennis, bowling, ball games, bicycling, etc.) when s/he is discharged;

— teach progressive muscle relaxation exercises & relaxed breathing techniques (such as natural childbirth type or hatha yoga type); see recommended references below;

— discuss with pt. the need for & value of daily quiet periods alone with self & for occasional long weekends in some leisure activity;

— investigate the possibility of biofeedback therapy to help pt. develop self control of muscular & nervous tension;

— consult with occupational & recreational therapy for appropriate relaxation suggestions (e.g. needlepointing, painting, learning to play a musical instrument, etc.);

— know that sedatives & tranquilizers are not effective in lowering BP & generally are not recommended for taking on a regular basis.

**3) Drug Therapy** The patient achieves a stable BP within physician-determined parameters; the patient is able to cope adaptively with drug's side effects, stating s/he realizes that the side effects are less dangerous than the effects of not taking the antihypertensive drug:

— know the expected & desired action of each drug given as well as the untoward effects to be observed & recorded; teach this to pt. & family; diuretics, sympathetic nervous system inhibitors and/or smooth muscle vasodilators may be given, but an attempt will be made to achieve sufficient reduction of BP with the lowest possible dosage of the fewest number of drugs, so it is important for the nurse to observe carefully & record accurately the pt.'s response to drug(s);

— question how the pt. feels & include the family's observations; side effects may include dry mouth, fatigue, diarrhea, depression, GI disturbances, drowsiness & others;

— observe for signs of potassium loss (calf or leg cramps, weakness, fatigue, mental confusion, apathy); check serum potassium level; for hypokalemia, pt. can eat foods high in potassium (raisins, prunes, orange juice, bananas, fish, leafy green veg.), can substitute KCL table salt for Na Cl, & doctor may order a potassium supplement; refer to NCPG #2:48, "Potassium Imbalance";

— if pt. is on a potassium-conserving diuretic, observe for signs of hyponatremia (lowered blood sodium: thirst, diminished sweating, fever, weakness, confusion) & hyperkalemia (weakness, numbness & tingling in extremities, slower pulse than normal, listlessness); pt. should **not** use a potassium-containing salt substitute, in this case;

— force fluids; dehydration from fever or hot weather enhances potency of hypotensive drugs;

— monitor & record TPR & BP when ordered & at other times to provide a guide or indication of drug effectiveness; note the pt.'s position (sitting, standing, lying down) & other pertinent variables (exercise, emotional reaction); keep the pt. informed of BP & let him assist in record keeping, so that s/he will feel informed & responsible for his own progress;

— watch for signs of orthostatic (postural) hypotension (dizziness, light-headedness); have pt. sit or squat down at first sign of weakness to prevent serious injuries from falls; teach pt. to assume a sitting position (after lying down) *slowly*, then a standing position while holding onto something, then a pause, before starting to walk;

— explore with pt./family any concerns or misconceptions s/he may have about taking medication daily for most of life; know that common feelings include embarrassment, guilt, fear of dependency, distrust of dosage amounts, disbelief & denial of need to take medications after s/he feels better, dismay over continuing cost of drugs; distress over unpleasant side effects & fear of sexual dysfunction which can occur as a side effect of some drugs; tell pt. that alternate drugs & dosages can be tried if side effects are intolerable, but that s/he must take some hypotensive drug(s) to keep BP under control;

— teach pt. to avoid over-the-counter cold remedies (which often contain vasoconstrictors) & aspirin compounds (which may contain caffeine) because these will interfere with their antihypertensive therapy;

— counsel & support pt. efforts to reduce or stop smoking; explain that nicotine is a vasoconstrictor & therefore increases the heart's work load; do not permit visitors to smoke in front of pt. & arrange for nonsmokers as pt. roommates;

— with the pt. & family, establish a medication routine that reduces the chance of error & forgetting; devise a simple schedule around the pt.'s work & sleep habits.

| | |
|---|---|
| 4) Psychosocial Adjustment | The patient accepts hypertension as a lifelong condition requiring continuing treatment; the patient expresses a firm commitment to actively participate in treatment program; the patient expresses fears, needs, and concerns to a receptive, empathetic professional person: |

— know that common fears & problems of hypertensives include: denial (of need to know about hypertension, of symptoms, of need to take medications when feeling good), excessive anxiety & tension, reluctance to be physically active, fear of missing too much work or failing to get a promotion because of repeated doctor appointments, misconceptions about hypertension disease, treatment & control; encourage pt./family to express these concerns; ask them what this condition will mean to pt. in terms of how s/he sees himself & lifestyle;

— assess pt.'s orientation to health, its value, pt.'s belief in prevention or only in cure; find out what pt. knows & determine what s/he needs & wants to know; help pt. identify own risk factors & the lifestyle changes s/he is willing to make to obtain control of condition;

— find out the possible obstacles to pt. keeping appointments, taking prescribed medications, adhering to diet, coping with stress, stopping smoking, exercising daily, & continuing to monitor own BP;

— answer questions, correct errors & gaps in knowledge, provide necessary information; evaluate & record what has been learned & determine what reinforcement & reminders will be needed;

— obtain a written or verbal commitment to comply with treatment regimen which pt. has had an opportunity to help plan & to express feelings & reactions concerning it; support & encourage pt.'s positive attitude & intentions to cooperate.

## Discharge Planning and Teaching Objectives/Outcomes

1) (Patient/Family/Significant Other) Can explain own specific pathology, its ramifications, what contributes to his disease process and the consequences of non-treatment.

2) Demonstrates an understanding of the what, why and when of total antihypertensive treatment program for own condition. Expresses willingness to assume responsibility for control of own BP and gives a commitment to follow treatment regimen faithfully.

3) Has received, read and understands written dietary instructions; can plan a typical day's menu and tell what is permitted or disallowed on the diet.

4) For each drug to be taken, know its purpose, schedule of dosage and untoward side effects to be observed and reported to doctor. Can express knowledge that his medications will help to keep his blood pressure down, only if s/he takes them continually on a regular basis, exactly as ordered, even after s/he feels completely well again.

5) Has received at least one descriptive pamphlet on hypertension, with doctor's approval, and has at least one community health resource person's name and number for getting further help and information (in addition to his doctor).

6) Can take own blood pressure accurately and knows when to notify doctor of results. (Get doctor's approval for teaching patient this technique.)

7) Has a follow-up appointment and promises (or contracts) to keep it.

**Recommended References**

"Breathing Techniques That Help Reduce Hypertension," by Sharon Dowdall. *RN*, October 1977:73–76.

"Diets: Low Sodium." *NCP Guide #3*:44, Nurseco, 1977.

"Guidelines for Educating Nurses in High Blood Pressure Control." High Blood Pressure Information Center, 120/80, National Institutes of Health, Bethesda, MD 20014.

"Helping The Hypertensive Patient Control Sodium Intake," by Martha Hill. *American Journal of Nursing*, May 1979:906–909.

"Helping Your Hypertensive Patients Live Longer," by Rosemary Maloney. *Nursing 78*, October 1978:26–34.

*High Blood Pressure (Hypertension)* and *Your Blood Pressure* (leaflets), American Heart Assn., 7320 Greenville Ave., Dallas, TX 75231.

"Potassium Imbalance." *NCP Guide #2*:48, 2nd. Ed., Nurseco, 1980.

"Promoting Patient Adherence," by Sue Foster and Deborah Kousch. *American Journal of Nursing*, May 1978:829–832.

"Protocol for Teaching Hypertensive Patients," by Ellen Mitchell. *American Journal of Nursing*, May 1977:808,809.

"Treating and Counseling the Hypertensive Patient," by Graham Ward et al. *American Journal of Nursing*, May 1978:824–828.

*Understanding High Blood Pressure*, Searle and Co., PO Box 5110, Chicago, IL 60680.

# The Patient with a Hysterectomy

**Definition:**   Hysterectomy is removal of the uterus: total (including tubes and ovaries) or sub-total (only the uterus), also known as a partial hysterectomy.

**LONG TERM GOAL:**   The patient will return to her optimum level of health and resume usual roles in home, family, community after a normal, short convalescence following safe, successful removal of uterus; the patient will accept and cope effectively with her altered body image and loss.

## General Considerations:

— Removal of the uterus may be done by abdominal or vaginal routes, depending on surgical diagnosis. Surgery may include A&P repair (anterior and posterior colporraphy—vaginal suture) for cystocele and rectocele (prolapses of bladder and rectum). Nursing care will vary accordingly, but principles re: restoration of normal function, prevention of complications, psycho-social adjustment remain essentially the same.

— **Preoperative nursing responsibility** is that for general abdominal surgery with the addition of a complete perineal prep and a cleansing douche, as ordered. Refer to NCPG #2:44, "General Preoperative Nursing Care." In addition, provide the patient with the information and reassurance she wants or needs re: hospitalization (usually a week or less), the operation, the expected post-operative course and convalescence. Nurses should be aware of what this operation means to patient so as to avoid inadvertent casualness or oversolicitude. Normal concerns include those of dying, of cancer, of disfigurement, of loss of femininity and sexuality, of pain, of loss of childbearing ability, of ability to cope or control destiny and of weight gain or other menopausal changes. The reactions and attitudes of husband, family and friends will affect the perceptions and the post-operative adjustment of the patient, as well as the length of convalescence.

— **Postoperative nursing responsibility** is that for general abdominal surgery (and is less complex for vaginal approach). Refer to NCPGs #2:41, 42, 43, "General Postoperative Nursing Care, Part A, Part B, & Part C." In addition, see NCPG #1:31, "Responses to Loss: the Grief and Mourning Process," and NCPG #2:29, "The Patient Experiencing a Body Image Disturbance." Most women under 40 can resume normal activities in a month and will feel quite like themselves or better in about two months. Older women in less ideal physical condition will need longer to regain strength and vitality.

**Specific Considerations, Potential Patient Outcomes, and Nursing Actions:**

1) General
   Abdominal
   Surgery
   Post-Op
   Measures

The patient will resume normal cardio-pulmonary function and fluid and electrolyte balance; the patient will be free of preventable complications:
— turn, cough, deep breathe & turn pt. Q2H;
— monitor & record TPR & BP according to standard postop routine until stable;
— monitor & record parenteral fluids; record I & O;
— administer antibiotics, vitamins & minerals, sedatives & analgesics as ordered; observe for untoward reactions;
— give food & fluids as tolerated when parenteral fluids are dc'ed & peristalsis returns;
— keep in low Fowler's or flat position to prevent increased intra-abdominal pressure; apply abdominal binder for additional support & comfort;
— give passive & active leg exercises at least Q4H; use elastic bandages for legs from ankle to groin & re-wrap Q8H; do not flex thighs sharply or place pt. in a high Fowler's position; leg dangling & progressive ambulation should be done as soon as surgeon permits.

2) Elimination

The patient will maintain adequate output and normal elimination will be restored after sutured area has begun sufficient healing:
— check indwelling catheter for patency & avoid dependent loops hanging below bed level;
— prevent bladder infection by sterile handling of tubes when disconnecting; use antibiotic ointment around meatus; obtain urine specimens from catheter with syringe & needle, using sterile technique;
— refer to NCPG #2:39, "Catheters: Indwelling Urinary";
— after catheter removal, check voiding Q4H; measure amt. voided; notify doctor if voiding frequent, small amts. or if unable to void in 6 hrs. if intake has been adequate; observe for signs of bladder infection;
— if rectocele has been repaired, a liquid low residue diet may be ordered to delay first defecation; then mineral oil laxatives and oil retention enemas are given to lubricate & ease movement without strain.

3) Perineal Care
   (for A-P Repair)
   & Dressings

The patient will heal with a minimum of discomfort and without infection:
— cleanse perineum with prescribed sterile solution twice daily & after each elimination; use heat lamp to help dry area & to promote healing;
— give sitz baths after sutures are removed for cleansing & comfort;
— for vaginal hysterectomy, encourage pts. to shower when able;
— check perineal pads to describe color, amt. & odor of drainage;
— for abdominal hysterectomy, reinforce dressing PRN; note amt. bleeding & report changes in pt. status.

4) Psychosocial
   Adjustment

The patient will adapt effectively to trauma of surgery, to her loss of uterus and altered body image; the patient will express growing confidence in ability to cope:

— teach & convince pt. that depression, weepiness, worry, helplessness & other seemingly unreasonable behavior are normal & expected; assure her that her ability to cope & remain in control will return in due course;
— help family & friends understand her need for repeated assurances of their love, concern & availability; encourage them to support her attractiveness & self-esteem; explore their cultural attitudes re: the female role in order to learn its probable effect on pt.'s perceptions:
— provide regular opportunities for talking, asking questions, expressing feelings & planning for future;
— re: intercourse, it is often helpful to say, "If you enjoyed it before, you will enjoy it afterwards," and vice versa; ending fears of pregnancy and relieving symptoms often improve intercourse but do not raise false hopes;
— provide copy of *After Hysterectomy, What?* (see ref.).

## Discharge Planning and Teaching Objectives/Outcomes

1) (Patient/Family/Significant Other) Knows what surgery has been done and what changes in herself to expect (menopausal symptoms, effects of hormonal therapy, weakness, fatigue, irritability & crying are customary) during convalescence.
2) Knows to avoid sexual intercourse, heavy lifting, vacuuming, pushing a full grocery cart, driving or prolonged sitting in a car, active sports or other "jarring" activities until doctor's approval (usually 4 to 8 weeks).
3) Knows that spotting and changing perineal pad twice daily is normal, but to report frank bleeding, increasing amounts of discharge or malodorous discharge promptly to doctor.
4) Understands and accepts responsibility for convalescence which may include: sitz baths, laxatives and medication for discomfort and rest, slow and moderate exercise with intermittent rest periods, a balanced diet and, for some, possible use of a girdle and support stockings. Knows that for some women, at least 9 weeks to three months may be required to "feel like themselves" again, depending on a variety of influencing factors (physical condition, mental attitude, increased age, attitude of family and friends, etc.).

**Recommended References**

*After Hysterectomy, What?* by Lindsay R. Curtis. ℅ Mallicote Printing, 509 Shelby St., Bristol, Tenn.
"Catheters: Indwelling, Urethral." NCP Guide #2:39, 2nd Ed., Nurseco, 1980.
"Easier Convalescence from Hysterectomy," by Margaret Williams. *American Journal of Nursing*, March 1978:438–440.
"General Postoperative Nursing Care, Part A, Part B, Part C." *NCP Guides* #2:41, 42, 43, 2nd Ed., Nurseco, 1980.
"General Preoperative Nursing Care," *NCP Guide* #2:44, 2nd Ed., Nurseco, 1980.
"Responses to Loss: the Grief and Mourning Process," *NCP Guide* #1:31, 2nd Ed., Nurseco, 1980.
"The Patient Experiencing a Body Image Disturbance," *NCP Guide* #2:29, 2nd Ed., Nurseco, 1980.

# The Patient with an Ileostomy

**Definition:**   Ileostomy is a surgically constructed bowel outlet on the abdomen, using the ileum.

**LONG TERM GOAL:**   The patient will recover from a successful ileostomy without preventable complications, returning to optimum health and usual roles in home, job, community after a normal convalescence; the patient will accept and cope realistically and adaptively to an altered body image and loss of normal elimination function.

### General Considerations:

— **Incidence:** There are approximately 1,500,000 ostomates in North America with nearly 100,000 new ostomy surgeries per year. Diseases which commonly necessitate ileostomy are chronic, advanced ulcerative colitis, familial polyposis, and Crohn's Disease (granulomatous colitis).

— **Ileostomy involves** the removal of the entire colon. The end of the ileum is brought out to the abdomen, forming a stoma. Fecal discharge is continuous or intermittent, but cannot be completely regulated and a collection bag is worn cemented to the skin. Some surgeons in a few large medical centers are now creating an internal pouch which retains ileal contents until the patient is ready to empty it at his convenience. The procedure, called a "continent" ileostomy, is still somewhat experimental since 1971, and is not recommended for obese patients or patients with regional ileitis or cancer.

— A proctectomy (removal of rectum) is usually also done. If not, the patient will have periodic mucus discharge from rectum and should be told this.

— **Nursing responsibilities** include (1) physical preoperative preparation of the patient with the usual measures for general abdominal surgery, i.e. operative and anesthesia consents, skin prep, nasogastric intubation, restriction of food and fluids, cleansing enemas, antibacterial medications and pre-anesthetic sedation. Refer to Nursing Care Planning Guide #2:44, "General Preoperative Nursing Care." (2) Provision for intellectual acceptance and emotional assimilation, preoperatively, by one or more of the following measures: have an enterostomal therapist, a mental health clinician or consultant, a qualified nurse or a selected ileostomate talk with patient, giving him an opportunity to ask questions, express concerns, seek reassurance, correct misconceptions and learn about the postoperative regimen. Normal fears are those of dying, of cancer, of pain, of disfigurement, of loss of sexuality, of inability to control body and what happens and of changed body image and self-concept. Actually sickness and disability have so changed the patient's lifestyle that an ileostomy is often a welcome release and afterward, most patients feel better than they have for years.

**Specific Considerations, Potential Patient Outcomes, and Nursing Actions:**

1) General
   Abdominal
   Surgery
   Postop
   Measures

The patient maintains adequate cardio-pulmonary, musculoskeletal and renal body functions; the patient is free of preventable complications of hemorrhage, infection, pneumonia and stomal damage; the patient is carefully monitored and free of complications of fluid loss, sodium and potassium deficit; the patient maintains adequate fluid and electrolyte balance:
— refer to NCPGs #2:41, 42, 43, "General Postoperative Nursing Care, Part A, Part B, Part C";
— monitor & record vital signs, CVP readings as ordered;
— monitor administration of parenteral fluids, electrolytes & vitamin supplements; refer to NCPG #2:46, "Intravenous Therapy: General Principles," NCPGs #3:48 & #3:49, "Fluids & Electrolytes, Part A & Part B";
— record I&O accurately; check urine output QH, recording specific gravity; watch closely for oliguria (reduced urine output);
— know that these pts. are especially vulnerable to fluid loss & electrolyte imbalance; watch for signs of sodium deficit (abdominal cramps, hypotension, rapid & thready pulse, apathy) & potassium deficit (weakness, paresthesias, faint irregular pulse, soft flabby muscles); refer to serum electrolyte reports & report promptly imbalances; see NCPG #2:48;
— turn, cough, & deep breathe pt. Q2H; have pt. exercise legs with each position change;
— keep nasogastric tube functioning & patent until peristalsis returns & tube is removed; record color & amt. drainage; provide oral hygiene Q2H;
— administer analgesics, sedatives, antibiotics as ordered.

2) Stomal Care

The patient will have adequate ileal drainage without blockage, leakage, skin irritation or odors; the patient will be able to care for own ileostomy:
— consult nearest local Enterostomal Therapist for information & help with pt.;
— observe & record color, amt. and consistency of ileostomy drainage; explain to pt. why drainage is watery & appliance needs frequent emptying to prevent pulling on the skin; empty when only 1/3 full;
— see NCPG #1:43, ". . . Changing a Temporary or Permanent Appliance"; note promptly & change a loosening or leaking appliance; prevent skin irritation with applications of plain tincture of benzoin & karaya gum rings or mixture;
— observe for peristomal monilia infection which is very common, especially in pts. on systemic antibiotics; look for erythematous center with a border of red papules; itching may be present; confirm with a culture; apply Mycostatin (R) Powder each time appliance is changed;
— observe & report stomal retraction or protrusion, peristomal skin irritation & infection; explain to pt. that stoma will continue to shrink in size for approx. 8 weeks as healing occurs & initial swelling subsides; tell pt. that some change in size & shape will also gradually occur over the first year; stress that because of this, it is necessary to measure stoma *each* time appliance is changed in order to fit the skin protective wafers & appliance *snugly* around stoma to prevent any leakage-caused skin excoriation;
— prevent & control humiliating odors by frequent emptying & rinsing of collection bag, by using deodorizing preparations

inside bag, by airing room after emptying bag, by using a room deodorant, & by having pt. take orally bismuth subgallate, N.F. for internal control of odor;

— encourage & provide means for pt. to assist & gradually assume care of own ileostomy as soon as s/he is physically & emotionally able; see NCPG #1:49, "Teaching Patients: General Suggestions," and NCPG #1:50, "Teaching Patients: Specific Plan for Skills & Procedures."

3) Nutrition    The patient will resume special diet as tolerated:

— gradually resume liquid, then soft, then regular consistency bland, low residue foods when nasogastric tube is removed; note pt. tolerance;

— introduce small amounts of each new food, noting intestinal reactions; teach pt. to do this at home;

— ask pt. to chew food completely, eating slowly to avoid blockage of ileum;

— know that severe gas pains are common; have pt. chew food with mouth closed, refrain from talking while eating, & avoid use of a straw for drinking liquids;

— teach pt. to avoid gas-forming foods such as beans, sauerkraut, cauliflower, cucumbers, onions, cabbage & carbonated drinks.

4) Psychosocial Adjustment    The patient will adapt realistically to an altered body image and self-concept; the patient will cope effectively with the loss of normal body elimination, accepting ileostomy and caring for it with confidence; the family expresses understanding and acceptance of patient's altered condition and provides emotional support to patient:

— be sensitive to behavioral cues: depression, silence, apathy, refusal to cooperate may indicate feelings of anger, grief, loss of self-esteem due to the shocking physical reality of the operation; refer to NCPG #1:31, "Responses to Loss: the Grief and Mourning Process";

— see NCP Guides on specific behaviors (#'s1:20-33); discuss pt.'s responses with pt./family & nursing staff & work together toward understanding & realistic plans of care; write approaches in care plan;

— arrange to have a successfully rehabilitated ostomate visit pt.;

— encourage pt. to touch stoma; refer to NCPG #2:29, "The Patient Experiencing a Body Image Disturbance"; help pt. to express feelings & to face the reality of the surgical experience; include the spouse or significant other in the pt.'s life so that discussions can be more beneficial: identify their concerns & correct misconceptions; recognize intimacy as a valued need & help them to discuss this openly, yet with sensitivity & understanding;

— provide pt./family/significant other with informational booklets from the United Ostomy Assn.; see recommended references.

## Discharge Planning and Teaching Objectives/Outcomes

1) (Patient/Family/Significant Other) States s/he knows basic facts re: diet, exercise, restriction of heavy lifting, medications (dosage, effects, untoward effects to be reported) returning to former job and activities.
2) Can describe the type of surgery and kind of stoma s/he has; demonstrates correct, safe confident care of ileostomy and appliance change.
3) Knows to report promptly to physician complications, abdominal cramps, vomiting, diarrhea, cessation of ileostomy drainage, pain, fever or other illness.
4) Has an identification card for wallet listing medications, routine of ileostomy care, the name and phone number of physician, and the next of kin to be notified in case of accident.
5) Has at least two weeks' ileostomy supplies and the name and address of local supplier for additional needs.
6) Has been evaluated for assistance (financial, vocational, social service disability, homemaker and home health care) and has received appropriate referrals.
7) Has the name and phone number of nearest local enterostomal theapist and/or community health nurse.
8) Knows how to handle *minor* episodes of constipation, diarrhea, and peristomal skin irritation.
9) Has received literature and information appropriate to needs and concerns; knows how to contact local ostomy association for further support services.
10) Has received the address of The United Ostomy Assn., Inc., 2001 Beverly Blvd., Los Angeles, CA 90057.

### Recommended References

"Basic Principles for Changing a Temporary or Permanent Appliance," *NCP Guide* #1:43, 2nd Ed., Nurseco, 1980.
"Fluids & Electrolytes, Part A: Fluids, Part B: Electrolytes," *NCP Guides* #3:48 & 3:49, Nurseco, 1977.
"General Postoperative Nursing Care, Part A, Part B, Part C," *NCP Guides* #2:41, 2:42, 2:43, 2nd Ed., Nurseco, 1980.
"General Preoperative Nursing Care," *NCP Guide* #2:44, 2nd Ed., Nurseco, 1980.
"Helping the Ileostomy Patient to Help Himself," by Jacqueline Lamanske. *Nursing 77*, January 1977:34–39.
"If the Ileostomy Is Continent, the Benefits Are Obvious," by Charlotte Isler. *RN*, April 1977:39–45.
"Intravenous Therapy: General Principles," *NCP Guide* #2:46, 2nd Ed., Nurseco, 1980.
"PostOperative Education For the Ileostomate," by Debra Broadwell and Suzanne Sorrells. *Ostomy Management*, May/June 1979:3–5.
"Potassium Imbalance," *NCP Guide* #2:48, 2nd Ed., Nurseco, 1980.
"Promoting a Positive Sexual Adjustment Following Ostomy Surgery," by Karla Rose-Williamson. *Ostomy Management*, May/June 1979:11–16.
"Responses to Loss: the Grief and Mourning Process," *NCP Guide* #1:31, 2nd Ed., Nurseco, 1980.
*Sex, Pregnancy and the Female Ostomate, Sex and the Male Ostomate, Ileostomy—A Guidebook*, and other literature. United Ostomy Assn., Inc., 2001 Beverly Blvd., Los Angeles, CA 90057.
"Teaching Patients: General Suggestions," *NCP Guide* #1:49, 2nd Ed., Nurseco, 1980.
"Teaching Patients: Specific Plan for Skills and Procedures," *NCP Guide* #1:50, 2nd Ed., Nurseco, 1980.
"The Patient Experiencing a Body Image Disturbance," *NCP Guide* #2:29, 2nd Ed., Nurseco, 1980.

# The Patient with a Mastectomy

**Definition:**   Excision of a breast: simple (breast only) or radical (breast with extensive lymph node dissection in surrounding tissues).

**LONG TERM GOAL:**   The patient will return to her optimum level of health and resume usual roles in home, family, community following a safe, successful breast removal and a suitable convalescence aimed at accepting her altered body image and loss; the patient will express optimism, self-confidence and a desire to live life fully and wholly again.

## General Considerations:

— **Incidence:** One in thirteen American women will develop breast cancer at some time in their life; over 100,000 new cases yearly, over 35,000 deaths yearly from breast cancer. More than 80% of lumps are first found by women themselves; most (over 80%) of these lumps are benign; high risk factors include previous cancer of breast and/or breast cancer in a close relative.

— **Cancer detection:** Nurses can assume an important role in early cancer detection by serving as specialized volunteers to teach breast self-examination in public health education programs. Training materials, films, and guidelines are readily available at the local ACS chapters. Nurses should remember and teach signs of possible breast cancer.

 B-breast mass, fixed, rigid, irregular;
 R-retraction, inverted nipple, "orange peel" skin signs;
 E-edema, swelling, change in size;
 A-axillary involvement of glands and nodes;
 S-sanguinous nipple discharge;
 T-tenderness.

— **Treatment:** Patients with breast disease are usually admitted for an excisional biopsy with frozen section and possible mastectomy. A simple lumpectomy may be indicated; a radical mastectomy may be needed, followed by (for metastases) radiation therapy, chemotherapy and/or hormonal therapy, oophorectomy, adrenalectomy, or hypophysectomy.

— **Preoperative nursing responsibilities** include:

 (1) Routine preop nursing care; refer to NCPG #2:44, "General Preoperative Nursing Care";

 (2) Specific teaching re: Hemovac, positioning, coughing and deep breathing exercises, dressing, pain relief & arm exercises;

 (3) Psychological and emotional care and counseling re: the information and reassurances that the patient needs and wants (hospitalization, the impending operation and probability of mastectomy, the postoperative course anticipated). Find out what the patient has been told and what is planned. Attempt to identify and resolve any distortions or misconceptions the patient may have. Do not force more information than the patient can tolerate or accept. Encourage patient to express her feelings and fears freely, even to cry. Normal and common fears include those of dying, of cancer, of disfigurement, of loss of sexuality, and of pain.

(4) Preparation of the family (or significant other), i.e. providing information, encouraging them to express their concerns and questions, helping them to understand the patient's feelings.

— **Postoperative nursing responsibilities** include:

(1) Routine postop nursing care; refer to NCPGs #2:41, 42, 43, "General Postoperative Nursing Care, Part A, Part B, Part C";

(2) Care of incision and arm: positioning, drainage, dressings; see below and refer to your hospital and surgeon's protocol;

(3) Psychological and emotional care to accept body image change and loss of breast as well as diagnosis of cancer with its implications; refer to NCPG #1:31, "Responses to Loss; the Grief and Mourning Process," and NCPG #2:29, "Body Image Disturbance."

(4) Teaching re: arm exercises, breast self-examination, prostheses and clothing selection; see below and refer to your own hospital's patient education program for mastectomy or develop one yourself in collaboration with American Cancer Society representative. Some of the information about prostheses and clothing will need to be provided by out-patient clinic or office nurse, by public health or visiting nurse, and/or by ACS volunteers in the weeks and months following the patient's discharge. The hospital staff nurse should be armed with referral names and numbers, with the addresses of local department stores or mastectomy boutiques that are prepared to help patient, and with literature on prostheses to use if requested.

— **Reach to Recovery Volunteers** are 3 years postop mastectomy patients verified by two doctors as being physically healed and psychologically adjusted. With the patient's physician request, the volunteer will visit in hospital or at home, bringing a kit of supplies, useful information, friendship, and strict confidentiality, free of charge.

— **The YWCA ENCORE National Program**, est. 1975, entails free, weekly group meetings of mastectomy patients for 30 min. "land exercises" and 30 min. "water therapy exercises" (shallow end of pool). A written consent form from the doctor is necessary.

## Specific Considerations, Potential Patient Outcomes, and Nursing Actions:

1) General Surgery Postop Measures

The patient will resume normal cardio/pulmonary/renal functions; fluid and electrolyte balance will be maintained and elimination patterns restored; the patient will be free of preventable complications:
— refer to NCPGs #2:41, 42, & 43;
— administer antibiotics, vitamin/mineral supplements, sedatives, etc. as ordered, observing & reporting untoward reactions;
— give fluids & food as tolerated when peristalsis returns;
— watch for bladder distention & constipation; take corrective measures needed.

2) Rest and Comfort

The patient will experience reduced discomfort and pain, less tension on the suture line; will be free of preventable immobility; the patient will maintain adequate ventilation, have clear lungs and will cough up bronchial secretions:
— position on back or unaffected side in semi-Fowler's position; use pillows & towels as cushions to keep elbow higher than shoulder, hand higher than elbow, joints flexed in functional position;
— turn, cough & deep breathe pt. Q2H, using gentle, firm support when moving affected arm; support chest during coughing;
— offer pain medication Q3-4H PRN; know that incisional pain lasts one to two weeks, but some pts. have intermittent pain or paresthesia at site for several weeks;

— give passive & active leg exercises Q4H until ambulatory; have pt. sit on side of bed, dangling legs with affected arm supported adequately for comfort; get pt. up to bathroom and begin progressive ambulation when surgeon permits.

| | |
|---|---|
| 3) Dressings & Drainage | The patient's incision will heal without infection or excessive bleeding; the patient will gradually assist with dressing changes until, by discharge, she can care for own wound site: |

— observe & record amt. & kind of drainage: handle Hemovac (or Vacu-Drain) & tubes carefully with aseptic technique; reinforce dressings as needed;

— report immediately excessive bleeding; check pulse & BP for significant change;

— encourage pt.'s acceptance & viewing of incisional site; gradually have pt. assist with dressing changes; teach pt. signs of infection to note & report to doctor, following discharge.

| | |
|---|---|
| 4) Arm Exercises | The patient's arm will be restored to full motion and usefulness; contractures, loss of function and stiffness will be controlled and muscle tone will be preserved: |

— make referral for physical rehabilitation, if formal program for mastectomy pts. is available in your hospital;

— have ACS Reach to Recovery Volunteer come in to teach exercises, if surgeon requests this in writing;

— refer to NCPG #1:45, "Arm Exercises for the Mastectomy Patient"; explain & demonstrate each exercise;

— stay with pt. while she does them for the first few days; use the opportunity to provide information, reassurance, encouragement & to assess any problems or answer any questions;

— involve a family member or friend to assist in encouragement of pt. & to help ensure faithfulness to exercise program in the weeks & mos. following discharge.

| | |
|---|---|
| 5) Psychosocial Adjustment | The patient will adapt effectively to the trauma of surgery, to her loss of breast and altered body image, to a cancer diagnosis and to the stress of an intensive rehabilitation regimen; the patient will express feelings openly and will gradually feel more confident and able to cope: |

— provide time to talk, to ask questions, to express feelings; remain with pt. for periods of time, even when pt. does not wish to talk; refer to NCPG #1:31 ". . . The Grief and Mourning Process;"

— allow the pt. to cry, to express anger, etc. in order to move steadily through grieving process without delay; help pt. to understand that crying spells, frightening dreams, helplessness & depression are not unusual & will pass;

— discuss her adjustment with family & friends; encourage them to support her attractiveness & self-worth; have them reassure the pt. that her femininity, sexuality & lovability are not affected by her appearance; help them to accept, to understand, & help pt.;

— consult surgeon re: information to be given pt. by whom; try to get a written request for a R-T-R Volunteer;
— teach pt. proper techniques of Breast Self-Examination; provide ACS pamphlet on topic (see references); help pt. accept fact that mastectomy pts. are higher risks & early detection of lump in other breast is her responsibility;
— accentuate the positive aspects of the pt.'s strengths, resources & value (to herself as well as others); identify & support the pt.'s desire to live fully again for as long as possible;
— evaluate emotional rehabilitation by time of discharge & make appropriate referrals for follow-up mental health care PRN; observe & assess pt. for signs of withdrawal, insomnia, depression, severe anxiety, helplessness & hopelessness.

## Discharge Planning and Teaching Objectives/Outcomes

1) (Patient/Family/Significant Other) Has been given a booklet or list of arm exercises and can demonstrate them accurately. Knows she should continue them for four to six months.
2) Has been given a pamphlet on Breast Self-Examination and can correctly demonstrate technique. Knows she must do this once monthly between periods, or at regular intervals.
3) Knows how to care for incisional area, dressings, etc. Knows what signs of infection (redness, swelling, increased drainage, odor, fever) to note and report promptly to doctor. Knows that complete healing should occur before fitting for a permanent prosthesis.
4) Knows that physical and mental exhaustion, probably related to stress reaction, will linger for several weeks; nevertheless, social visits and resumption of activities of daily living should be gradually undertaken.
5) States she knows how to prevent lymphedema (or swollen arm): sleeping or sitting with affected arm elevated; keeping skin clean, healthy, free of injuries and minor infections; using talcum powder instead of anti-perspirants which clog pores; exercising arm faithfully; refraining from using tight bracelets or carrying heavy handbags or packages; wearing gloves for house and yard work; and avoiding extremes of heat or cold.

**Recommended References**
"Arm Exercises for the Mastectomy Patient," *NCP Guide* #1:45, 2nd. Ed., Nurseco, 1980.
"Breast Cancer: Confronting One's Changed Image," a series of articles by various authors. *American Journal of Nursing*, September 1977:1430–1436.
"Breast Cancer—Helping the Mastectomy Patient Live Life Fully," by Joanne Tully and Beatrice Wagner. *Nursing 78*, January 1978:18–25.
"Breast Examination Practices," by Ellie Turnbull. *American Journal of Nursing*, September 1977:1450, 1451.
"Breast Self-Examination," by Doris Burger. *American Journal of Nursing*, June 1979:1088, 1089.
*Breast Self-Examination, Reach To Recovery* (pamphlets for patients). American Cancer Society, Inc., 521 W. 57th St., New York, NY 10019.
"General Postoperative Nursing Care, Part A, B, & C," *NCP Guides* #2:41, 42, 43, 2nd. Ed., Nurseco, 1980.
"General Preoperative Nursing Care," *NCP Guide* #2:44, 2nd. Ed., Nurseco, 1980.
"Responses to Loss: the Grief and Mourning Process," *NCP Guide* #1:31, 2nd. Ed., Nurseco, 1980.
"The Patient Experiencing a Body Image Disturbance," *NCP Guide* #2:29, 2nd. Ed., Nurseco, 1980.

of restrictions: if pt. objects strongly, s/he may be better off if allowed to do a few things for self, eg. feeding; use judgment;

— explain all procedures & use of equipment, inc. system of alarms on monitor; disturb pt. as little as possible; no bed baths for at least 48 hrs., wash face & hands & give mouth care PRN; prevent loud noises, excessive talking or bustling activity within hearing range of pt.;

— assess impact of a family member visiting & regulate visits accordingly;

— after first 48 hours, pt. should cough & deep breathe, turn from side to side Q2H; give passive ROM exercises QD (see NCPG #1:47); don't use knee gatch or isometric exercises; check with Dr. if pt. can sit in chair; if yes, remember that chair rest means *rest*, not activity; provide chair with a firm seat, leg & arm rests; as activity is increased, monitor tolerance; check on EKG changes;

— avoid any sudden physical exertion or straining; place things within easy reach of pt.;

— monitor responses to progressive diet regimen; restrict caffeine & sodium.

3) Pain

The patient will experience no pain or will experience minimal pain and be relieved of pain by medication, rest, and reduced anxiety level:

— pt. is usually sedated for first 48 hours to ensure rest; check BP, P, & R before medicating; hold medication if R less than 12-14/mins.; check BP and P 20 mins. after medicating, to determine effect of them, if any; notify Dr. if medication depresses vital signs &/or if pain persists;

— stay with pt. during severe pain, to give emotional support; observe for non-verbal signs of pain; some pts. may deny discomfort or be afraid to ask for meds; explain that heart will rest better if pain is absent; check with pt. at least Q2H to ask if s/he has discomfort;

— assess & chart type, intensity & location of pain.

4) Psychosocial Adjustment (to Loss of Usual Body Functioning)

The patient will verbalize own feelings/concerns about the illness/loss and will begin to feel some control over own life:

— pt. &/or family may go through initial stages of Grief & Mourning; shock, denial, disbelief (see NCPG #1:31, "Responses to Loss"); allow them to use any of these defense mechanisms to cope with this current situation;

— you can help modify the loss by presenting *a calm, supportive attitude; by acknowledging pt.'s feelings,* explaining that these are normal, temporary & will diminish; *by including pt. in planning* & carrying out own care within limits of his condition; *by finding out who are pt.'s sources of emotional support,* eg. spouse, children, friend, confidante, & permitting them to visit, so as to decrease pt.'s feelings of isolation; *by flexing visiting hours; & by accepting pt. where s/he is:*

angry, upset, uncooperative, wanting to talk about death (see NCPG #1:27, "Dealing with Impending Death"), & not avoiding pt.; know that any angry feelings are not meant for you personally, but are expressions of rage in response to the current loss; clergy availability often appreciated, but no visits without pt.'s OK;

— point out signs of progress (eg. "Your pulse is slower now, and that's a good sign."); know correlation of serum enzymes to clinical course & use judgement in interpreting them to pt.;

— the experiencing of a loss may temporarily increase the cardiac work load; be alert to signs of this (distended jugular veins, changes on monitor, ashen skin, color changes in lips & nail beds); monitor changes carefully; provide physiological support: eg. meds, $O_2$, etc.; notify Dr. PRN;

— determine if pt. has had any other significant losses in last 6 months & his way of coping with them; help pt. to use his usual coping methods; assess how s/he perceives the loss, eg. a loss of usual role functioning? job? etc.; provide information re: his prognosis & usual functioning & what s/he will be able to do physically; help pt. focus on what s/he will be able to do, not on what has been lost; see NCPG #2:35, "Crisis Intervention";

— modify hospital environment by bringing pt.'s things into room; provide a calendar, clock, small radio, ad lib; include pt. in planning daily care & schedule; have pt. make as many decisions as possible (this gives pt. back some control over own life);

— when pt. is transferred from the CCU/ICU to the floor, it will be normal for him to feel anxious over loss of security of the critical care unit; i.e. monitors, constant surveillance, low pt.-nurse ratio; help modify this by advance planning: a nurse from new unit should come & visit pt. before transfer, reinforce that move is a sign of progress, & that feelings of anxiety & insecurity are usual, expected & temporary.

## Discharge Planning and Teaching Objectives/Outcomes

1) (Patient/Family/Significant Other) Can discuss the impact of MI on patient's heart and activity level, diet and emotional state.
2) Can state the need for ongoing self-assessment and accept the reduced monitoring that will occur in non-CCU environment.
3) Refer to this section in NCPG #2:15, "The Patient with an MI: Convalescent Phase."

### Recommended References

"Central Venous Pressure Line (CVP)." NCP Guide #2:40, 2nd Ed., Nurseco, 1980.
"Crisis Intervention: Adaptation to General Nursing." NCP Guide #2:35, 2nd Ed., Nurseco, 1980.
"Dealing with Impending Death." NCP Guide #1:27, 2nd Ed., Nurseco, 1980.
"Drugs: Cardiac." NCP Guide #2:37, 2nd Ed., Nurseco, 1980.

"Diets: Low Sodium." NCP Guide, #3:44, 1977.

"Four Steps for Better Cardiac Care in the E.R.," by Margaret Miller and Linda Lazure. *Nursing 78,* August 1978:40–43.

"Helping Spouses of Critically Ill Patients," by Christine Breu and Kathy Dracup. *American Journal of Nursing*, January 1978:50–53.

"Intravenous Therapy: General Principles." NCP Guide #2:46, 2nd Ed., Nurseco, 1980.

"Memory Bank for Critical Care," by Gary Ervin. Pacific Palisades, CA.: Nurseco, 1979.

"Physical Assessment, Part D: Auscultation." NCP Guide #4:50, Nurseco, 1978.

"Potassium Imbalance." NCP Guide #2:48, 2nd Ed., Nurseco, 1980.

"Pump Failure Following Myocardial Infarction: An Overview," by Sue Foster and Kathleen Canty.
*Heart and Lung*, March–April 1980:293–297.

"Responses to Loss: the Grief and Mourning Process." NCP Guide #1:31, 2nd Ed., Nurseco, 1980.

"Right Ventricular Infarction," by Joanne Sunquist, Frank Mikell, Gary Francis and Morrison Hodges.
*Heart and Lung*, July–August 1980:706–710.

"Sleep and the Cardiac Patient," by Judith Hemenway. *Heart and Lung*, May–June 1980:453–463.

"The Patient Experiencing a Body Image Disturbance." NCP Guide #2:29, 2nd Ed., Nurseco, 1980.

"What Every Nurse Should Know About EKGs," by M. Van Meter and P. Lavine. *Nursing 75*, May 1975:37–43 (and subsequent issues).

# The Patient with a Myocardial Infarction: Convalescent Phase

**LONG TERM GOAL:** The patient will achieve maximum physiologic, emotional, and functional rehabilitation within the limits of the cardiac disability while retarding the progress of arteriosclerosis and preventing congestive heart failure.

## General Considerations:

— **Nursing responsibilities:** health teaching of patient and family assumes a very large role; assessment of their existing knowledge of the disease process, medications, diet, and Rx is necessary in order to plan appropriate teaching. Reinforcement of what was taught since admission will be necessary; much may have been forgotten due to the emotional upset.

— The patient's best insurance against future problems is an adequate knowledge of the disease and healing processes, adherence to dietary and medical regimens, and a healthy adaptation to the loss. An understanding of the concept of cardiac rehabilitation programs and relating the needed information to the patient/family is an important nursing responsibility.

— Review NCPG #2:14, "The Patient with a Myocardial Infarction: Acute Phase," and the recommended references.

## Specific Considerations, Potential Patient Outcomes, and Nursing Actions:

1) Rest and Activity

The patient will cooperate in a routine that will minimize cardiac work load; will maintain muscle tone and skin integrity; will establish a daily, regular and gradual exercise program:

— amt. of activity allowed will depend on the pt.'s cardiac status & tolerance; check with Dr. for permitted exercise & activity levels; be specific about amt. & type of exercises & activity pt. may do; continue with ROM exercises QD;

— elicit pt.'s feelings re: exercise/activity program; stress importance of adherence to regimen for optimum rehabilitation;

— discuss regimen with family; use opportunities to discuss pt.'s normal activity & occupation & the modifications which may need to be made after discharge;

— encourage pt. to walk but advise it be done daily, slowly increasing time & distance; avoid extremes in temperature & walking against the wind;

— have pt. acknowledge the need to rest after meals & before any exercise;

— space activities so as to alternate work & rest;

— explain that exercise stress testing will be done after the myocardium heals so that ongoing activity levels can be determined.

2) Diet

The patient will accept dietary modifications and assist in the planning of daily menus:

— elicit pt.'s feelings about the dietary restrictions; permit pt. to verbalize whatever s/he wishes; if s/he denies the

importance of the diet, do not support the denial, but support any efforts s/he makes to accept & work with the diet;
— assess pt.'s understanding of the importance of the dietary regimen to maintenance of health; reinforce & provide information PRN;
— reinforce teachings of dietician; if one not available, teach the elements of the dietary regimen & reinforce on a daily basis; include family; have pt. make up daily menus, check them & correct PRN;
— help pt. understand need for potassium supplements (either prescription or by orange juice twice a day);
— help pt. make adjustments in usual home diet; discuss need to reduce intake of caffeine (tea, coffee, soft drinks), alcohol, & salt;
— encourage pt. to eat 3-4 meals daily, avoiding large meals & eating quickly.

3) Health Teaching

The patient will be able to communicate an understanding of the disease and healing processes; will verbalize rationale, actions, and possible side effects of all medications s/he is taking:
— elicit pt.'s feelings re: illness & prognosis; correct any misconceptions; provide as much information as you & the pt. feel s/he wants to know; give pt. pamphlets from American Heart Association; reinforce & discuss your teaching with pt. on a daily basis; include family;
— discuss risk factors of overweight, smoking, drinking, stress, diet;
— provide pt. with a written list of medications, their actions & side effects; ensure that s/he knows importance of taking as ordered; if on Digitalis, teach pt. to take own pulse; refer to NCPG #2:37, "Drugs: Cardiac";
— reinforce the four basic principles of maintaining optimum health as outlined under "General Considerations";
— refer to NCPG #1:49, "Teaching Patients: General Suggestions," & #1:50, "Teaching Patients: Specific Plan for Skills & Procedures";
— instruct pt. as to what signs & symptoms necessitate calling his Dr.

4) Psychosocial Adjustment (Continued Adaptation to the Loss)

The patient will mourn adaptively; will recognize activities, functions, and/or roles that have not been lost; will have self-esteem and self-confidence about his ongoing life style:
— know that adaptive responses will be: asking questions about the loss, alternately denying & accepting the loss; answer all questions as best you can; if you don't know answer, find someone who can help; be honest, don't give false reassurance; do not focus on what has been lost, but do focus on what pt. can & will be able to do;
— include pt. in planning daily schedule; allow him to make as many decisions as possible; give him as much control over

his life as you can; when pt. wishes, have personal things brought from home;
— review NCPG #1:31, "Responses to Loss."

## Discharge Planning and Teaching Objectives/Outcomes

1) (Patient/Family/Significant Other) Can verbalize knowledge of the disease and healing processes involved in MI.
2) Has a written list of all medications being taken home; knows actions and possible side effects; knows how and when to take medications and obtain refills; can take own pulse.
3) Knows and accepts dietary restrictions; can identify restricted foods and plan daily menus; has a written diet plan to take home.
4) Knows prescribed activity level, and is aware of the relation of activity and energy expenditure to functional capacity of the heart. Has a plan for expending energy conservatively throughout the day, interspersed with adequate rest periods. Knows to avoid strenuous activities, climbing stairs, driving a car, or air travel until Dr. OKs. Has a written activity/exercise regimen to take home.
5) Is aware of signs and symptoms of problems and knows to report them to Dr. Has Dr. clinic appointment for follow-up treatment.
6) Can identify at least two potential stress-provoking situations and has at least one alternative for dealing with them.
7) Can discuss feelings related to loss of usual body functioning and/or usual roles and/or job. Asks questions related to these losses and has tentative plans for modifying lifestyle to adjust to them.
8) Has an ID card in wallet with diagnosis, medications, Dr.'s name, phone number, and information re: nearest relative.

**Recommended References**

"After a Coronary." "Heart Attack." and other patient-teaching pamphlets available free from American Heart Association, 44 E. 23rd St., New York, NY 10010 (or a local chapter).
"Drugs: Cardiac." NCP Guide #2:37, 2nd Ed., Nurseco, 1980.
"Diet: Fat-Controlled, Low Cholesterol." NCP Guide #4:43, Nurseco, 1978.
"Rehabilitation of the Cardiac Patient, the Effects of Exercise," by Michael Dehn. *The American Journal of Nursing*, March 1980:435–439.
"Rehabilitation of the Cardiac Patient, Progressive Exercises to Combat the Hazards of Bedrest," by Elizabeth Winslow and Therese Weber. *The American Journal of Nursing*, March 1980:440–445.
"Rehabilitation of the Cardiac Patient, Bridging the Gap Between Inhospital and Outpatient Care," by Anne Devney. *The American Journal of Nursing*, March 1980:446–449.
"Rehabilitation of the Cardiac Patient." Improving Compliance with an Exercise Program," by Jean Hoepfel-Harris. *The American Journal of Nursing*, March 1980:449–450.
"Postmyocardial Infarction Syndrome," by Ann Hirsch. *The American Journal of Nursing*, July 1979:1240–1241.
"How Long Does Grief Go On?" by Mary Jo Klepser. *The American Journal of Nursing*, March 1978:420–421.

# The Patient with a Nephrectomy

**LONG TERM GOAL:**   The patient will recover from the surgery free of preventable complications.

## General Considerations:
— Indications for surgery are tumors (most are unilateral and malignant), irreparable damage, or kidney donation.
— Normal renal function can be maintained by a single healthy kidney.
— Nursing responsibilities include adequate pre-op preparation (see NCPG #2:44), including assuring patient that s/he can function perfectly well with only one kidney, and close post-op monitoring of vital signs and fluid balance.

## Specific Considerations, Potential Patient Outcomes, and Nursing Actions:

1) Prevention of Complications   The patient will be closely monitored for early signs of impending complications; will receive prompt intervention to control complications:
  — review NCPGs #2:41, 42, 43, "General Post-Op Care";
  — know that colicky-type pain may occur (due to passage of clots down ureter); it is usually short-lived; medicate PRN;
  — know that common complications include hemorrhage (due to slippage of a ligature from a renal vessel), pneumothorax (a rupture of diaphragm may sometimes occur because of close proximity to surgery), abdominal distention (occurs frequently due to a reflex paralysis of intestinal peristalsis);
  — check vital signs & dressings frequently for signs of frank hemorrhage; if renal suture has slipped, hemorrhage can be rapid & fatal; call surgeon at slightest suspicion;
  — auscultate chest for adequate breath sounds, especially on operative side; know early warning signs of pneumothorax (sudden, sharp, chest pain; dyspnea; weak pulse; acute anxiety & restlessness; diaphoresis; decreased breath sounds); notify surgeon at once; place pt. in semi-Fowler's position & give $O_2$;
  — know that an NG tube may be used to prevent abdominal distention; auscultate abdomen for sounds at least Q4H (pt. may be NPO until they return); when able, clamp tube, start on fluids & increase as tolerance permits; use rectal tube or Harris flush PRN (to relieve flatus, distention).

2) Fluid Balance   The patient will maintain an adequate fluid balance; will be monitored for early signs of kidney malfunction:
  — with adequate intake, urinary output should be at least 500 cc/day; observe, measure & chart amt., color, odor, concentration, content, specific gravity;

— foley catheter is vital to protect remaining kidney from infection & to monitor output; do not irrigate without surgeon's order; anchor catheter to pt. to prevent pull & tension on it; pin to bed sheet so that a direct line with some give goes to drainage bag; prevent kinking, compression or bending of tube, so urine will not pool in bladder &/or back up into kidney; refer to NCPG #2:39, "Catheters: Indwelling Urethral";

— know signs & symptoms of fluid imbalance; read NCPG #3:48, "Fluids";

— maintain fluid intake as Dr. orders; measure & chart accurately; explain to pt. that adequate intake is important as vehicle to excrete wastes, chemicals, & electrolytes, & to prevent urinary stasis & infection.

3) Psychosocial Adjustment (to Loss of a Body Part)

The patient will respond adaptively to the loss of a kidney; will move through the grief and mourning process:

— know what behaviors are considered adaptive/maladaptive for this process & support accordingly; see NCPG #1:31, "Responses to Loss: the Grief & Mourning Process";

— be aware that this loss will be experienced just as intensely by renal donors as by pts. with renal tumors or damage; staff sometimes "neglects" the donor pt. because s/he is free of disease but in reality, this pt. needs a great deal of emotional support, especially if pressure has been put on pt. to be a donor.

## Discharge Planning and Teaching Objectives/Outcomes

1) (Patient/Family/Significant Other) Knows s/he should be as active as possible but refrain from lifting heavy objects for 1 year post-op.

2) Knows importance of adequate fluid ingestion and indicates a willingness to maintain this at prescribed level.

3) Understands the necessity of going through grief and mourning process over loss of kidney (for good mental health); knows what to expect re: feelings of sadness, change in self-image, etc.

**Recommended References**

"Catheters: Indwelling Urethral." NCP Guide #2:39, 2nd Ed., Nurseco, 1980.

"Fluids and Electrolytes, Part A: Fluids." NCP Guide #3:48, Nurseco, 1980.

"General Postoperative Care, Parts A, B, C." NCP Guides #2:41, 42, 43, 2nd Ed., Nurseco, 1980.

"General Preoperative Care." NCP Guide #2:44, 2nd Ed., Nurseco, 1980.

"Potassium Imbalance." NCP Guide #2:48, 2nd Ed., Nurseco, 1980.

"The Renal Donor," by Delores Schumann. *American Journal of Nursing*, January 1974: 105–110.

"Responses to Loss: the Grief and Mourning Process." NCP Guide #1:31, 2nd Ed., Nurseco, 1980.

# The Patient with a Pacemaker

**Definition:**  A pacemaker is an electrical device used to provide stimulation to the ventricles so that consistent cardiac contraction is produced.

**LONG TERM GOAL:**  The patient will be able to resume and maintain usual activities and roles, being aware of the limitations and precautions associated with this cardiac assistive device.

**General Considerations:**
— **Artificial pacing** is used for bradycardia that does not respond to drug treatment, 2nd or 3rd degree A-V block, bilateral bundle branch block, &/or ventricular dysrhythmias where overdrive of the ventricles is necessary to suppress ectopic sites. Pacemakers have both prophylactic and therapeutic uses.
— **Temporary pacing** is utilized during diagnostic evaluation of Bundle of His studies, tachydysrhythmia studies, as well as to increase the heart rate in patients with coronary artery disease so the added stress on the heart can be studied. In addition, it is used prophylactically in patients with A-V block receiving an anesthetic, in postoperative cardiac surgery patients, on patients undergoing surgery for permanent pacemaker insertion or battery replacement, on patients with electrolyte imbalance such as hyperkalemia, and in treatment of pre–renal azotemia in renal failure. Temporary pacemakers are inserted transcutaneously, by transvenous or transthoracic approach and are generally controlled by an external device.
— **Permanent pacing** is always therapeutic and is used to treat patients that are symptomatic and have complete A-V block, certain patients with asymptomatic A-V bloc, sick sinus syndrome (includes symptomatic bradycardia, sinoatrial block, sinoatrial arrest, and bradycardia-tachycardia syndrome), hypersensitive carotid sinus syndrome, and in tachydysrhythmias unresponsive to drugs.
— Permanent pacemakers are inserted through a transvenous, transmediastinal or transthoracic approach and are controlled by a battery-operated internally placed device. Placement of the triggering electrode is in the ventricular epicardium. Batteries used to maintain pacemaker function need to be recharged or replaced periodically. The time frame varies from several weeks to several years, depending on the type of power source. Familiarize yourself with type of power sources and replacement/recharge schedules.
— **Pacemaker rates vary:**
   • *fixed pacing:* rate is predetermined, fixed and independent of the electrical activity of the heart.
   • *synchronous pacing:* stimulates ventricular contraction after each atrial beat; is preset and functions if spontaneous cardiac activity does not occur.
   • *demand pacing:* QRS stimulus-inhibited pacemaker which comes into function at a preset rate if spontaneous cardiac activity does not occur.

- *sequential pacing:* two electrodes pace the atrium and/or ventricle when either sinus rhythm or normal conduction does not occur.
— **Nursing responsibilities** include familiarization with the type of pacemaker used, rationale for use, monitoring patient's physical and emotional status, and teaching patient/family about device and its expected outcomes.

**Specific Considerations, Potential Patient Outcomes, and Nursing Actions:**

1) Pre-Operative Preparation: Fear/ Apprehension

The patient is able to express his fears and apprehensions regarding a surgical procedure and dependence on a pacemaker:
— answer all questions honestly, do not give false reassurance; explain procedure & pacemaker function; if pt. does not ask questions or express feelings, help him to do so (eg. "Many people are upset at the thought of being dependent on a pacemaker. How do you feel?"); explain that an implanted pacemaker should not interfere with usual living patterns; provide a used pacemaker for pt. to handle if available and if pt. desires;
— refer to NCPG #2:44, "General Preoperative Care."

2) Prevention of Complications

The patient will be monitored closely for early signs and symptoms of complications; will be free of preventable complications:
— refer to NCPGs #2:41, 42, 43 "General Post-Op Care: Support of Pulmonary, Cardiovascular, Renal, and Auxiliary Functions";
— if pt. has had a thoractomy, refer to NCPG #1:19, "The Patient with a Thoractomy" & NCPG #1:34, "Chest Tubes & Bottles: Water-Seal Drainage";
— cleanse & protect skin around venipuncture site; apply antibiotic ointment at least Q8H;
— know & observe for signs of *perforation of ventricle* (muffled heart sound, low BP with a narrow pulse pressure, cyanosis, restlessness, increased CVP); *cardiac tamponade* hemorrhage into the pericardium (faint heart sounds, narrow pulse pressure, high CVP with low BP, distended neck veins, dyspnea, cyanosis, shock): *infection* (fever, malaise); report to surgeon; an elevated temp. may mean pt.'s tissues are rejecting the unit;
— observe for signs of dizziness, local hematoma, air emboli, pneumothorax;
— a Hemovac will usually be in place at site of pacemaker; explain purpose to pt.;
— start ROM exercises on 2nd PO day; shoulder on operative side is especially prone to immobility; give pain meds. ½ hr. before ROM: refer to NCPG #1:47, "ROM Exercises."

3) Pacemaker Functioning

The pacemaker will function as regulated; early signs of malfunctioning will be detected.
— know exactly which type of pacemaker is being used: what kind of rate? Check with surgeon & read literature from manufacturer; if pacemaker is bipolar type (has a "spare"), pt. is reassured there is a back-up system;

— check BP & pulse (rate, volume, regularity) as often as you judge pt.'s condition dictates; a pulse variation of more than 5/ min. or any erratic beats should be reported to surgeon; read cardiac monitor to detect conduction defects; note pacemaker artifact on reading;
— monitor and analyze ECG readings;
— check pacemaker threshhold Q8 hours.

4) Psychosocial Adjustment

The patient will express feelings indicative of a sense of well-being and independence:
— discuss pt.'s living patterns with him, exploring the effects, if any, a pacemaker will make on them; encourage both positive and negative feelings; usual ones involve dying, dependency, disability. restrictions; explain that these are expected and temporary;
— teach pt. to take own pulse, to know signs of early pacemaker malfunctioning; battery failure usually causes pulse slowdown; if timing mechanism fails, pulse speeds up;
— explain that a pacemaker does not correct the underlying problem causing the conduction defect; give reasons for this & emphasize need to adhere to prescribed cardiac regimen;
— when pt. ready, arrange for another pacemaker pt. to visit.

## Discharge Planning and Teaching Objectives/Outcomes
1) (Patient/Family/Significant Other) Can take own pulse and states will do so at least twice/day; will keep written record for doctor. Knows acceptable variations for own pacemaker and to report unacceptable ones to doctor, as well as episodes of syncope, blackout spells, and chest pain. Knows battery will need to be changed on periodic basis, 18-24 months.
2) Knows to avoid close proximity to high frequency electrical equipment, automobile engines, lawn mowers, snowmobiles, microwave ovens. Is aware s/he cannot receive treatment with electrocautery or high frequency dentist drills.
3) Carries a card indicating s/he has an implanted pacemaker.
4) Verbalizes an understanding of permissible activity (will vary with patient's age and condition).
5) Has appointment for visit with doctor/clinic; is aware that such visits will be necessary at least 3/year.

#### Recommended References
"Chest Tubes and Bottles: Water Seal Drainage." NCP Guide #1:34, 2nd Ed., Nurseco, 1980.
"General Post-Op Care, Parts A, B, C." NCP Guides #2:41, 42, 43, 2nd Ed., Nurseco, 1980.
"General Pre-Op Care." NCP Guide #2:44, 2nd Ed., Nurseco, 1980.

*Living with Your Pacemaker,* available from: American Heart Association, 44 East 23rd St., New York, N.Y. 10010—or your local Heart Association.

"Patients with Pacemakers," by Hannelore Sweetwood. *Nursing 77,* March 1977:44–51.

"Protecting Patients with Temporary Transvenous Pacemakers" by Cecile E. Hammond. *Nursing 78,* November 1978:82–86.

"The Patient with a Thoractomy." NCP Guide #1:19, 2nd Ed., Nurseco, 1980.

"What Patients Need to Know About Pacemakers," by Mary Manwaring. *The American Journal of Nursing,* May 1977:825–830.

# The Patient with Parkinson's Disease

**Definition:** Parkinson's Disease is caused by pathological changes in the basal ganglia of the cerebrum. This produces a deficiency of dopamine which affects body movement and muscle tone.

**LONG TERM GOAL:** The patient (and family) will accept this disease, adapting to necessary limitations and a lifestyle incorporating a balanced program of exercise, medication and optimal health habits; the patient will preserve functional capabilities and prevent severe disabilities and deformities for as long as possible.

## General Considerations:

— **Signs and symptoms:** slow, steady progressive development; tremors (alternating muscular flexions & contractions) that are maximal at rest & decrease with movement, yet are absent during sleep; voluntary muscle rigidity or stiffness; restlessness or jitteriness; slowness of movement with periods of frozen action; weakness & easy fatigability; altered facial expressions (pain-like) with open mouth, rotating eyes, increased lacrimation and salivation; slurred, monotonous, low tone of voice; and occasional fever, sweating, pallor, incontinence, and constipation.

— **Treatment** includes: medications to control symptoms, exercise to lessen complications of impaired mobility and good health habits generally advocated for older persons (since P.D. is more common over 60).

## Specific Considerations, Potential Patient Outcomes, and Nursing Actions:

1) Susceptibility to Hazards (Related to Impaired Mobility)

The patient will be free of preventable injuries and infections; the patient will express less fear of falling, less embarrassment, and more self-confidence in ability to help self safely:

— provide good lighting in bathrooms, hallways, closets & near bedsides; install handrails & non-skid floors;

— arrange for firm mattress on low bed with overhead trapeze or pull rope; provide canes, walkers, wheelchairs PRN; use straight backed arm chairs;

— have pt. use firm soled shoes instead of slippers; "freezing" & difficulty starting movement are common, so provide gentle, encouraging help with first move; teach pt. to begin walking with a short step backwards, then to move forward on the extended leg, placing heel on floor before toes; gait training & practice sessions may be needed;

— offer your arm, hand or rail for pt. to hold, rather than supporting pt.'s waist or arm, thereby unbalancing pt.; have pt. swing arms naturally when possible & look straight ahead; avoid excessive help & reassure to assuage fear of falling; avoid sense of haste or impatience & control onlookers when possible to reduce pt.'s tension & embarrassment which worsen situation;

— allow extra time for trips to bathroom, dining room, therapy or other activities; plan to arrive early & leave late to reduce crowding, haste or curious gawkers;

— observe proper body alignment in bed, chair or when walking; see NCPG #2:45, "Hazards of Immobility";

— keep skin clean, dry & free of irritations or pressure areas; provide emollient skin massages to arms, legs, face, neck, shoulders & back muscles; change position every hour; use cushions at pressure points;

— know that impaired throat & chest movements predispose a pt. to excessive salivation, dysphagia, congestion & respiratory infection; provide accessible tissues for frequent expectoration; help pt. to turn, cough & deep breathe regularly; use side-lying positions or elevate head of bed to prevent choking; maintain adequate fluid intake; recognize early signs of illness & get prompt, medical treatment.

2) Activity/ Exercise

The patient will retain muscle and joint flexibility; the patient will be free of preventable complications of muscular atrophy, weakness, contracture, stiffness and degenerating postural deformities for as long as possible:

— arrange for daily physical therapy (heat, massage, exercise, gait training);

— plan & conduct a regular program of daily, medical–approved exercise with the assistance of both pt. & family member; refer to NCPG #2:32, "Exercises for Patients over 65"; encourage several short daily walks;

— give full range of motion exercises to pts. on bed rest or limited ambulation; see NCPG #1:47, "Range of Motion Exercises"; give pt. soft balls to squeeze periodically in hands;

— insist on pt. standing up at least a dozen times daily with feet wide apart; have sitting pts. cross & uncross legs periodically;

— arrange for daily activities (social, recreational, occupational) which require use of voice, hands, arms or legs and reduce social isolation; (ex. sporting events, card-playing, jacuzzi sessions with someone, etc.)

— ask pt. to read aloud 15 min. twice daily to strengthen & improve voice & breathing coordination, pronunciation & volume; have pt. sing in shower or join an amateur singing group, if feasible.

3) Diet and Medications

The patient will maintain a balanced nutrition appropriate to medication type; the patient will have symptoms reduced with suitable dosage levels and drug combinations; the patient will recognize, understand & accept undesirable but common side effects while preventing serious complications and untoward effects:

— refer to NCPG #2:38, "Drugs: Parkinson's Disease;"

— administer high carbohydrate, moderate protein, low fat diet that is ample in residue and fluids; serve portions that are

small (four or five feedings a day) because of slow eating patterns, difficulty swallowing & need to improve drug absorption & effectiveness;
— give medications with meals; observe & record all signs & symptoms, side effects, tolerance & drug effectiveness carefully & completely;
— limit alcohol intake which can antagonize drug effects;
— help overweight pts. to reduce in order to facilitate regulation of effective drug dosage levels & to reduce probabilities of cardiovascular complications.

4) Elimination    The patient will maintain normal elimination patterns utilizing measures to regulate and control incontinence or constipation:
— teach pt. importance of diet & exercise to maintain elimination patterns;
— refer to NCPGs #2:39, "Catheters: Indwelling Urethral," #2:03, "The Patient for Bladder Retraining," & #2:04, "The Patient for Bowel Retraining."

5) Clothing    The patient will dress self with minimal difficulty; overheating will be prevented:
— while sweating is a symptom of P.D., drug therapy reduces this, so overheating in hot weather is a dangerous possibility; recommend light, cotton clothing; teach pt. to avoid unnecessary exertion & to remain indoors on hot, humid or smoggy days; avoid chilling by fans or air-conditioners;
— advise use of shoes without laces, pants with loose fitting legs, dresses with front zippers, velcro closures or hooks instead of buttons when possible.

6) Psychosocial Adjustment (to Loss of Usual Body Functioning)    The patient feels free to voice any negative feelings about his disease and the limitations it imposes; the patient understands and accepts the reality of condition and tries to live as normal a life as possible within the therapeutic regimen and limitations of disease's progressive degeneration; the patient responds adaptively to loss of independence and to an altered body image and self-concept:
— explore with pt./family feelings & fears related to Parkinson's Disease with its limiting effects; common fears include those of falling, of choking, of loss of control over their lives, of dependency & worthlessness, of embarrassment & social isolation related to altered facial expressions, speech patterns & body movements;
— encourage pt. to continue pursuit of work, hobbies, sports, recreational, social & civic activities previously enjoyed, for as long as possible; advise discretion & judgment to prevent fatigue, tension, frustration, injuries, & infections which will worsen symptoms;

— consult with ministers, social workers, mental health workers & the pt.'s friends & family to assist you & pt. to progress effectively in the desired medical treatment-rehabilitation program;

— see NCPG #1:31, "Responses to Loss," NCPG #1:26, "The Patient Experiencing Depression," and NCPG #1:28, "The Patient Experiencing Fear."

## Discharge Planning and Teaching Objectives/Outcomes

1) (Patient/Family/Significant Other) States understanding of basic facts of Parkinson's Disease; has received and read *A Manual For Patients With Parkinson's Disease.*

2) Has been provided with a written set of instructions re: medications, activities, exercises, prevention and early control of complications, infections, constipation, drug therapy side effects; has appointment for medical follow-up; has expressed intent and willingness to carry out recommendations.

3) Has been evaluated for assistance (financial, social security disability, vocational, convalescent hospital or home health care) and appropriate referrals have been made to local and state agencies.

4) Has address of national and local Parkinson's Disease Association; has information re: additional community resources and services (senior citizens, self-help groups, meals or transportation help, etc.); has at least one community health worker's name and number (besides own doctor) in order to get additional help and information when necessary.

### Recommended References

*A Manual For Patients With Parkinson's Disease,* by Drs. Richard Sweet and Fletcher McDowell. The American Parkinson's Disease Association, 147 E. 50th Street, New York, N.Y. 10022.

"Catheters: Indwelling Urethral," *NCP Guide #2:39,* 2nd Ed., Nurseco, 1980.

"Drugs: Parkinson's Disease," *NCP Guide #2:38,* 2nd Ed., Nurseco, 1980.

"Easing Adjustment to Parkinson's Disease," by Frances Fischbach. *American Journal of Nursing,* January 1978:66–69.

"Exercises for Patients Over 65," *NCP Guide #2:32,* 2nd Ed., Nurseco, 1980.

"Hazards of Immobility," *NCP Guide #2:45,* 2nd Ed., Nurseco, 1980.

"Helpful Tips You Can Give Your Patients with Parkinson's Disease," by Cindy Gresh. Nursing 80, January 1980:26–33.

"Range of Motion Exercises," *NCP Guide #1:47,* 2nd Ed., Nurseco, 1980.

"Responses to Loss: the Grief and Mourning Process," *NCP Guide #1:31,* 2nd Ed., Nurseco, 1980.

"The Patient Experiencing Depression," *NCP Guide #1:26,* 2nd Ed., Nurseco, 1980.

"The Patient Experiencing Fear," *NCP Guide #1:28,* 2nd Ed., Nurseco, 1980.

"The Patient for Bladder Retraining," *NCP Guide #1:03,* 2nd Ed., Nurseco, 1980.

"The Patient for Bowel Retraining," *NCP Guide #1:04,* 2nd Ed., Nurseco, 1980.

# The Patient with Phlebitis

**Definition:** Phlebitis is inflammation of the wall of a vein; thrombophlebitis is phlebitis with thrombus formation; phlebothrombosis is thrombus formation with vein inflammation.

**LONG TERM GOAL:** The patient will recover from the acute condition, and will adhere to a regimen designed to prevent future occurrences.

## General Considerations:
— **Causes:** Can occur after direct trauma, as an extension of an adjacent infection, the result of continuous pressure (aneurysm, tumor, O.R. table straps, knee gatch, bed rolls), as a complication of varicose veins, or may result from any condition that promotes venous stasis (pregnancy, prolonged immobility, obesity, congestive heart failure).

— **Occurrence:** May occur in either superficial or deep veins. More common in women (70%) than in men, since women take birth control pills and get pregnant. Phlebitis and thrombophlebitis occur most often in leg veins; may occur after prolonged use of an IV site (12 hours + ) or due to irritating IV solutions. Phlebothrombosis occurs most often post-op, and is often mistaken for muscle ache due to wearing flat slippers.

— **Symptoms:** May be mild, and include stiffness, soreness, edema, redness and heat over affected area, pain in upper posterior calf or dorsiflexion of foot (Homan's sign). May lead to severe pain on pressure, marked tenderness over affected area, often with slightly elevated temp. and pulse.

— **Nursing responsibilities** include eliciting patient cooperation in adhering to prescribed treatment, alleviating patient's anxiety, and teaching preventive health measures.

## Specific Considerations, Potential Patient Outcomes, and Nursing Actions:

1) Impaired Circulation, Pain & Anxiety

The patient will adhere to prescribed therapeutic regimen; will experience minimal pain and anxiety:
— keep pt. on bed rest, with leg elevated (with pillows & raising foot of bed) to degree ordered by Dr.; check with Dr. as to amt. of activity pt. permitted (will vary); know & share with pt. that bed rest is usually continued until all symptoms are gone for several days;
— provide heat (as ordered) via K-pad, hot soaks, or heat cradle;
— apply elastic stockings or bandages as ordered (they compress superficial veins & prevent stasis); remove for 15 mins. BID; inspect skin underneath for irritation, tenderness;
— avoid rubbing or massaging leg because of risk of dislodging thrombus; if clot does move to lung, may cause subtle or blatant symptoms (sub-sternal pain, dyspnea, rapid & weak pulse, fever, cough); see NCPG #2:22, "Pulmonary Embolus";

— provide pain relief with meds. PRN; if pt. on anti-coagulants, ensure they are given on time; see section on these drugs in NCPG #2:37, "Cardiac Drugs";

— assess pt.'s anxiety level; know that providing information is often an effective way of reducing anxiety; assess pt.'s perception of expected outcomes of treatment, knowledge of condition & provide information PRN; share any signs of positive change with pt.

2) Surgical Intervention

The patient can state the rationale for surgery, and has realistic expectations re: outcomes; the patient will be free of preventable complications:

— assess pt.'s knowledge of surgery rationale, procedure & outcomes; correct misconceptions PRN;

— know that surgery may be done when pt. is unable to take anticoagulants, when there is a high risk of pulmonary emboli, or when there is severely compromised venous drainage; procedures include ligation of femoral veins or inferior vena cava to prevent thrombi from breaking off & becoming pulmonary emboli, & venous thrombectomy to remove clot;

— see NCPGs #2:41, 42, 43, 44, "Pre- and Post-Op Care."

3) Health Teaching

The patient can state rationale of, and will adhere to, prescribed regimen designed to present venous stasis and possible recurrences of acute condition:

— prevent dehydration (which leads to concentration of blood) by ensuring an adequate fluid intake;

— prevent venous stasis by avoiding prolonged periods of immobility (should get up & walk for 5 mins. at least Q2H); if on a long automobile/plane trip, arrange to do walking as above;

— avoid prolonged pressure, particularly under knees (as might occur with long periods of sitting in one position in chair), by elevating feet, uncrossing knees, changing position at least Q2H;

— work with pt. to develop an exercise plan that will fit in with his daily activities at home/work; include getting up and walking, or wiggling toes, ankles & legs for at least 5 mins Q2H; if pt. leads a sedentary lifestyle, explain that unusual physical activity should be avoided;

— explain importance of maintaining all facets of prescribed medical regimen as a preventive measure.

## Discharge Planning and Teaching Objectives/Outcomes

1) (Patient/Family/Significant Other) Knows pre-disposing factors of phlebitis and to avoid those within his control, e.g. prolonged periods of immobility, unusual physical activity, prolonged pressure on a vein, dehydration, trauma, bruising.

2) Knows when to wear elastic stockings, including wearing time, but to avoid wearing tight garters, girdles or any other constricting clothing.
3) Can demonstrate an exercise routine which includes walking, moving toes in shoes, elevating legs for 5 minutes Q2H, elevating legs above head 2-3 times QD; knows to do this daily.
4) Can verbalize medications to be taken at home, including actions, dosages, and possible side effects.
5) Knows early signs and symptoms of phlebitis and to report them stat to doctor/clinic.

**Recommended References**

"Drugs: Cardiac." NCP Guide #2:37, 2nd Ed., Nurseco, 1980.
"General Pre-Op Care." NCP Guide #2:44, 2nd Ed., Nurseco, 1980.
"General Post-Op Care, Parts A, B, C." NCP Guides #2:41, 42, 43, 2nd Ed., Nurseco, 1980.
"How Patient Education Can Reduce the Risks of Anticoagulation," by Karen Moore and Barbara J. Maschak. *Nursing 77*, September 19:24–29.
"The Patient With Pulmonary Emboli." NCP Guide #2:22, 2nd Ed., Nurseco, 1980.
"Thrombophlebitis in Pregnancy," by Jo Ellen S. Nyman. *American Journal of Nursing*, January 1980:91–93.
"Low-Dose Heparin Therapy," by Susan Lee Chamberlain. *American Journal of Nursing*, June 1980:1115–1117.

# The Patient with a Prostatectomy

**LONG TERM GOAL:**   The patient will recover from surgery free of preventable complications, and will return to usual roles (state what they are).

**General Considerations:**
— **Indication** for surgery is prostatic enlargement, which impedes urinary bladder outlet, preventing free passage of urine; usually a slow but continuous process.
— **Incidence:** 50-65% of men over 50 have some prostatic enlargement: 80-88% are benign, 12-20% malignant; is second only to skin cancer as most common malignancy in men.
— **Symptoms:** may be of *urinary infection and stasis* (dysuria, frequency, nocturia); of *urethral obstruction* (hesitancy, decreased size and force of urinary stream, retention, hematuria, dribbling); of *renal complications* (urethral dilation; hydronephrosis, renal infection).
— **Types of surgical approaches:** choice depends on age and condition of patient, size and location of gland enlargement:
   1) *Transurethral resection* (TUR/TURP): a closed procedure done in cysto, in which a loop of wire connected to a cutting current is rotated through a cystoscope, shaving off prostate at bladder orifice. Advantages: no incision, safer surgical risk, short hospital stay, potency maintained. Disadvantages: recurrent obstruction can develop; delayed bleeding may occur.
   2) *Suprapubic:* abdominal incision into bladder. Advantages: more complete removal of obstructing gland with exploration for Ca. lymph nodes. Disadvantages: urinary leakage around suprapubic tube onto skin, control of hemorrhage difficult, convalescence prolonged and uncomfortable.
   3) *Perineal:* incision in perineum. Advantages: direct anatomical approach allows hemostasis under direct vision, less incidence of shock, low mortality rate. Disadvantages: high post-op incidence of impotency, urinary incontinence, and rectal damage.
   4) *Retropubic:* low abdominal approach, but not into bladder. Advantages: easier control of hemorrhage with shorter period of convalescence. Disadvantages: increased incidence of inflammation of pubic bone.
— **Nursing responsibilities** include preparing the patient for surgery (see NCPG #2:44), both emotionally and physically (ensuring adequate bladder drainage and hydration) and helping patient cope with physical/emotional adjustments post-op.

**Specific Considerations, Potential Patient Outcomes, and Nursing Actions:**
1) Urinary      The patient will be free of urinary stasis; will be adequately hydrated:
   Elimination      — irrigate catheters only as ordered by physician; check urethral catheter for signs & symptoms of obstruction or bright blood;

— explain to pt. that urge to urinate is due to bladder spasm & not to twist or pull on catheter;
— keep catheters & tubes patent, free from kinks, uncoiled;
— assess pt.'s complaint of abdominal pain to see that drainage tubing is free of obstruction prior to giving analgesic &/or antispasmodic;
— give 2-3000 cc's/day of oral fluids, unless contraindicated; assess pt. for signs of adequate hydration or dehydration; see NCPG #3:48, "Fluids & Electrolytes";
— measure I&O accurately & chart; record times of urination after catheter is removed until an acceptable voiding pattern is established;
— inspect urine for amt. of bleeding, clots, pieces of tissue immediately post-op & Q2H; chart findings;
— refer to NCPG #2:39, "Catheters: Indwelling Urethral."

**2) Prevention of Complications**
The patient will be monitored for detection of early signs and symptoms of post-op complications; will be free of preventable complications:
— know that complications & nursing actions specific to the surgery are:
  • *for TUR:* if pt. complains of sharp pain, report to surgeon stat; bladder may be perforated; may need Foley with large inflated bag to apply pressure to control bleeding;
  • *for suprapubic:* tube goes directly to bladder, thus give meticulous asceptic attention to area around it; if order given to irrigate tube, use separate irrigation set & aseptic technique; protect skin from irritation of urine by covering with Karaya gum paste or other effective ointment; change dressing as ordered by surgeon; may have penrose drain;
  • *for perineal:* no rectal temps, tubes or enemas; change dressings only as ordered by surgeon; report any redness, oozing or extreme pain at incision; use double-tailed T binder to secure dressings without causing pressure on incision; heat lamp & sitz baths may be ordered to promote healing, decrease discomfort;
  • *for retropubic:* penrose drain usually present; change dressing as ordered;
— observe closely for shock, hemorrhage; see NCPG's #2:41, 42, 43, "General Post-Op Care."

**3) Bladder Control**
The patient will regain bladder control; will be able to empty bladder adequately:
— pt. may have a degree of loss of bladder control & urinary frequency; explain to pt. that this is a common occurrence post-op, that regaining control is a gradual process, & that he can expect dribbling to continue for a period of time;
— check with doctor re: perineal exercises for pt.; this routine can be helpful:
  • instruct pt. to tense perineal muscles by pressing buttocks together, hold position as long as possible, then relax;

should be done 10-20 times/hour; continue with exercises until full control is achieved;

— explain to pt. that regaining bladder control after surgery is a gradual process & that he can expect dribbling to continue for a period of time.

| | |
|---|---|
| 4) Psychosocial Adjustment (to Loss of Usual Body Functioning) | The patient will verbalize feelings related to any changes in bladder control and/or sexual functioning:<br>— be aware that these pts. may be experiencing decreased self-esteem, embarrassment, fear of impotence, &/or depression due to loss of, or change in, functioning (sexual &/or bladder control); explain that these are usual, expected feelings following prostatectomy; see NCPG #1:31, "Responses to Loss";<br>— spend time with pt. each day, encouraging him to verbalize his feelings; assess where pt. is in moving through the grief & mourning process; include spouse/significant other in discussion, if pt. wishes; point out any signs of recovery and progress;<br>— know that pt. may be aggressive & exert independence as reaction to sexual role interference; see NCPG #1:20, "The Patient Manifesting Aggression." |

## Discharge Planning and Teaching Objectives/Outcomes

1) (Patient/Family/Significant Other) Knows to be physically active but to avoid strenuous exercise and heavy lifting for at least three weeks post-op.
2) Knows what is an adequate fluid intake for him, the importance of maintaining this level, and verbalizes a willingness to comply.
3) Knows signs and symptoms of urinary infection, decreased urinary flow or obstruction, and to report to doctor at once; knows to report signs of bleeding.
4) Knows what to expect in terms of bladder control, sexual role functioning, and feelings related to any dysfunction.

**Recommended References**

"Catheters: Indwelling Urethral." NCP Guide #2:39, 2nd Ed., Nurseco, 1980.

"Fluids and Electrolytes, Part A: Fluids." NCP Guide #3:48, Nurseco, 1977.

"General Postoperative Care, Parts A, B, C." NCP Guides #2:41, 42, 43, 2nd Ed., Nurseco, 1980.

"General Preoperative Care." NCP Guide #2:44, 2nd Ed., Nurseco, 1980.

"Responses to Loss: the Grief and Mourning Process." NCP Guide #1:31, 2nd Ed., Nurseco, 1980.

## The Patient with Pulmonary Edema

**Definition:** A life-threatening situation wherein fluid from over-congested lungs has leaked through the capillary walls into the alveoli.

**LONG TERM GOAL:** The patient will return to a stable physical condition, adhering to prescribed medical regimen designed to prevent recurrences.

### General Considerations:
— Pulmonary edema is an extreme form of left-sided heart failure: a weakened left ventricle is unable to push out sufficient blood to the body, while the right side continues to pump blood into the lungs, resulting in lung congestion. If uninterrupted, this process leads to increasing respiratory difficulty, a significant drop below normal in $pCO_2$ and $pO_2$, and respiratory failure. The patient is literally drowning in his own secretions.

— **Symptoms** usually appear at night after patient has been recumbent for a few hours (related to reabsorption of edema from legs) and include dyspnea, orthopnea, restlessness, anxiety, cough. May lead to an acute attack with cyanosis, cold/moist hands, rapid, moist/gurgling respirations, severe apprehension, cough productive of pink, frothy sputum, rapid pulse.

— **Treatment** is urgent and is aimed at reducing venous return to the heart and increasing left ventricular outflow.

— **Nursing responsibilities** include constant, alert monitoring of patient's physiological and emotional status throughout the crisis, and intervening as necessary to maintain patient's equilibrium.

### Specific Considerations, Potential Patient Outcomes, and Nursing Actions:

1) Cardio/Pulmonary Function

The patient will be oxygenated adequately; will resume normal breathing pattern; will maintain a patent airway; will have a more effective circulation compared to admission status:

— place pt. in an upright sitting position, with feet & legs down (to prevent further lung engorgement & to favor pooling of blood in dependent area of body);

— give $O_2$ to relieve hypoxia & dyspnea; mask or nasal catheter deliver highest concentration; pts. often tolerate mask poorly due to fear of suffocation;

— rotating tourniquets may be used to trap blood in the extremities (comparable to withdrawing 1 liter of blood): tourniquets are applied to 3 extremities at once & rotated Q15 mins.; may rotate clockwise *or* visa versa, but *always in same direction;* direction should be recorded (or make a diagram) & known to all care givers (to avoid confusion or dangerous error); tourniquets should be tight enough to block venous return but not cut off arterial circulation; check distal pulses after applying; to remove, continue rotating Q15 mins. until all are off (to remove all at once would overload the heart); electric tourniquets may be used; if so, read operating instructions carefully;

— explain to pt. that his extremities will be swollen, mottled & uncomfortable due to engorgement with venous blood, & that this will disappear after removal of tourniquets;

— know that phlebotomy may be carried out (as a means of decreasing venous pressure & volume of circulatory blood); 200-500cc is usually withdrawn (often results in dramatic improvement);

— observe & chart rate & quality of *pulse* (full, bounding, weak, regular), *respirations* (shallow, rapid, slow), *skin appearance* (color, turgor, moistness), *cough* (productive of what, dry);

— keep accurate I&O; insert Foley catheter as ordered; keep pt. NPO until ordered otherwise;

— CVP line may be used; see NCPG #2:40, "CVP Line";

— observe for signs of potassium depletion (see NCPG #2:48, "Potassium Imbalance"); check pt.'s blood gas levels (normal pH: 7.35-7.45; $pCO_2$: 40-45mm Hg, $pO_2$: (varies with pH)mm Hg.—about 90mm Hg); see NCPG #3:40; "Acid-Base Balance."

2) Drug Therapy   The patient will experience a degree of relief from acute symptoms; the patient will verbalize the names, rationale, actions and possible side effects of prescribed drugs to be taken after discharge:

— know that meds. are a chief line of treatment; pt. may be digitalized (to increase cardiac output); diuretics are given to produce diuresis; aminophylline often given to dilate bronchi;

— observe pt. response to meds.; watch for signs of intolerance; read NCPG #2:37, "Drugs: Cardiac";

— know that toxic effects of digitalis can cause dysrhythmias such as bigeminy, paroxysmal atrial tachycardia, A-V block; monitor pt.'s EKG carefully;

— maintain an open IV line as route for emergency drugs, but do not allow over-infusion;

— give morphine judiciously; keep on hand for emergency use.

3) Anxiety and   The patient will maintain anxiety feelings at a sub-panic level; the patient will express decreased anxiety/fear, increased
   Fear   relaxation:

— stay with pt. during critical phase (to provide comfort & ensure safety); remain calm & confident while around pt. & family;

— tell pt. what is happening to him, including types of Rx & rationale; explain that he can expect some relief from symptoms within a few hours; share any signs of progress, eg. favorable changes in respirations, pulse, output, blood gases;

— give morphine as ordered (to reduce restlessness, apprehension, anxiety); chart effect on anxiety & respirations;

— know that these pts. often feel "closed in" & "suffocating"; open windows PRN, keep bed curtains open; use light bed covers; do not "crowd" pt.;

— see NCP Guides #1:22, "Anxiety," & #1:28, "Fear."

## Discharge Planning and Teaching Objectives/Outcomes

1) (Patient/Family/Significant Other) Knows warning signs and symptoms of pulmonary congestion (paroxysmal, nocturnal dyspnea; cough; restlessness; anxiety) and knows to seek medical help when these appear.

2) Has written list of medications, actions and side effects to take home; can verbalize the importance of taking medications to prevent future attacks.

3) Knows permissible amount of daily fluids, and to avoid ingestion of a large amount at one time. If prescribed, can select foods and menus for a sodium-restricted diet; can state acceptance of need and value of following diet.

4) Knows to weigh self daily as a check on excess fluid retention, and to report excess to doctor/clinic.

5) Knows to sleep with head of bed elevated approximately 10 inches and to avoid excessive and/or sudden physical exertion.

**Recommended References**

"Acid-Base Balance." NCP Guide #3:40, Nurseco, 1977.

"Catheters: Indwelling Urethral." NCP Guide #2:39, 2nd Ed., Nurseco, 1980.

"Central Venous Pressure Line." NCP Guide #2:40, 2nd Ed., Nurseco, 1980.

"Drugs: Cardiac." NCP Guide #2:37, 2nd Ed., Nurseco, 1980.

"Intravenous Therapy: General Principles." NCP Guide #2:46, 2nd Ed., Nurseco, 1980.

# The Patient with a Pulmonary Embolus

**Definition:**   Lodgement of an embolus in one or more of the pulmonary arteries.

**LONG TERM GOAL:**   The patient will recover from the acute episode and will internalize a health-maintaining regimen designed to prevent future occurrences.

**General Considerations:**
- **Origin:** majority arise from deep veins in legs or pelvis, some from right atrium; fewer from irritating IV solutions, fractures of large bones. Most emboli are thrombi, but may also consist of air (from IVs), fat (from fractures of large bones), tumors, or amniotic fluid.
- **Predisposing factors:** most important is **venous stasis** resulting from conditions involving slow venous return to heart, eg. immobility, varicosities, fractures, congestive heart failure, phlebitis. Other factors include hypercoagulability of blood, atrial fibrillation, obesity, injury, or change of muscle wall of vein.
- **Symptoms** may be sudden or with gradual onset and depend on *size* of embolus and *area* of pulmonary artery involved; large embolus at bifurcation of pulmonary artery produces a sense of impending doom, sudden sub-sternal pain, dyspnea, rapid and weak pulse, shock, syncope, sudden death; in right or left pulmonary artery: dyspnea, mild sub-sternal pain, weakness and tachycardia, fever, cough, hemoptysis; in terminal pulmonary arteries: cough, hemoptysis, pleurisy-like pain.
- **Early detection** is difficult because of subtlety of symptoms, and often stems from a nurse's suspicions and observations of subtle changes in TPR, BP, diaphoresis, chest pain, cough. Patients at high risk for pulmonary emboli include those with prolonged immobilization, heart disease, abdominal surgery, obesity, stroke, previous history of emboli, phlebitis, severe trauma, and women who take birth control pills and smoke cigarettes.
- **Prognosis:** approximately 38% die within two hours of onset; with careful observation and intervention, the remainder recover. Clots usually disappear spontaneously in about 50% of those patients who survive 2-3 weeks.
- **Nursing responsibilities** include knowing if patient is in high risk group, observing for and being alert to early signs and symptoms, and providing intensive nursing care to return patient to a state of physical and emotional equilibrium.

**Specific Considerations, Potential Patient Outcomes, and Nursing Actions:**

1) Impaired Circulation & Respiratory Function

The patient will experience acute symptomatic relief; will be monitored closely for changes in physiological status; will have adequate cardiopulmonary functioning restored:
- place pt. on strict bed rest; avoid use of knee gatch or pillow under knees; elevate head of bed to relieve SOB; give $O_2$ as ordered; have intubation equipment ready for emergency use;

— have emergency drugs & CVP line available (see NCPG #2:40);
— give IVs as ordered; pt. usually put on anti-coagulant therapy (see NCPG #2:37, "Drugs: Cardiac"); ensure they are given accurately & on time; observe & chart pt.'s response;
— apply elastic stockings; remove for 15 mins. BID; inspect skin for tenderness & irritation;
— monitor vital signs as often as you judge necessary; auscultate chest for breath sounds, rales; record I&O accurately;
— assess & chart pt.'s response to interventions; as pt.'s condition stabilizes & improves, check with Dr. re: ROM exercises (see NCPG #1:47) & other activity permitted;
— know that surgery may be scheduled; procedures include ligation of femoral vein or inferior vena cava (to prevent additional emboli from migrating to heart & pulmonary artery); or open heart surgery with cardiopulmonary bypass (to remove emboli from pulmonary artery);
— if pt. scheduled for surgery, explain rationale, procedures, expected outcomes; assess what information pt. wants & needs to know; review NCPGs #2:41, 42, 43 on pre- & post-op care, &#4:06, 07 on Cardiac Surgery.

2) Anxiety    The patient will verbalize anxiety; will experience no more than a moderate level of anxiety:
— some pts. with sudden pulmonary emboli may feel a sense of doom; stay with pt. to ensure comfort & safety; ask pt. to close eyes & visualize self breathing easily & comfortably; repeat PRN;
— clarify situation for pt.; explain that most cases of embolism respond to anti-coagulant therapy; when pt. ready, provide information on drug actions, rationale, etc.;
— share signs of measurable progress with pt., eg. vital signs, CVP readings, decrease in symptoms; let pt. know what s/he can expect from Rx in terms of mobility, relief of symptoms, etc.;
— inform pt. of all procedures & rationale before carrying them out;
— review NCPGs #1:22 & 28, "Anxiety" & "Fear."

3) Health Teaching    Refer to this section in NCPG #2:19, "Phlebitis."

**Discharge Planning and Teaching Objectives/Outcomes**
1) (Patient/Family/Significant Other) Can verbalize an understanding of venous stasis and its relationship to embolus formation; knows to avoid predisposing factors such as sitting with legs crossed, immobility, padding under popliteal area, tight straps around knees, etc.
2) Can do full ROM and knows to do these at least BID; knows to get up and ambulate for 5-10 mins. Q2H, except during night, but during all other hours, including when riding in an automobile or airplane.

3) Knows when to wear elastic stockings, including wearing time, and to avoid wearing tight garters, girdles or any other constrictive clothing.
4) Knows what medications to take, and when; has a written list of medications, including actions and possible side effects.
5) Knows early signs of impending pulmonary emboli (cough, dyspnea, pain or muscle ache in chest) and thrombophlebitis (stiffness, soreness, redness over affected area) and to report these to the doctor or clinic at once.

**Recommended References**

"Central Venous Pressure Line." NCP Guide #2:40, 2nd Ed., Nurseco, 1980.
"Drugs: Cardiac." NCP Guide #2:37, 2nd Ed., Nurseco, 1980.
"General Post-Op Care, Parts A, B, C." NCP Guides #2:41, 42, 43, 2nd Ed., Nurseco, 1980.
"General Pre-Op Care." NCP Guide #2:44, 2nd Ed., Nurseco, 1980.
"The Patient Experiencing Anxiety." NCP Guide #1:22, 2nd Ed., Nurseco, 1980.
"The Patient Experiencing Fear." NCP Guide #1:28, 2nd Ed., Nurseco, 1980.
"The Patient Undergoing Cardiac Surgery: Pre-Op and Post-Op." NCP Guides #4:06, 07, Nurseco, 1980.
"The Patient with Phlebitis." NCP Guide #2:19, 2nd Ed., Nurseco, 1980.
"Pulmonary Embolism: Don't Overlook These Subtle Warnings," by Jane B. Falotico. *RN*, February 1979:47–52.
"Range of Motion Exercises." NCP Guide #1:47, 2nd Ed., Nurseco, 1980.

## The Patient with Renal-Ureteral Calculi

**LONG TERM GOAL:**   The patient will recover from acute phase free of preventable complications, and will adhere to prescribed medical regimen designed to prevent complications.

### General Considerations:

— **Predisposing conditions:** renal infection, urinary stasis, prolonged periods of immobility, dehydration, genetic factors, hypercalcemia and hypercalciuria (may be caused by hyperparathyroidism or excessive intake of milk or vitamin D), high mineral content in water, vitamin A deficiency.

— **Symptoms:** dull ache in back or flank with increasing amounts of blood and pus in urine; pain may become acute and colicky. N&V may be present; perspiration often present as stone passes. Renal stones cause an increase in hydrostatic pressure, distending renal pelvis and proximal ureter leading to bladder. Symptoms of urinary tract infection include chills, fever, dysuria, hematuria, dull back/flank pain.

— Stones may be found anywhere in the urinary tract, from kidney to bladder; vary from gravel size to that of an orange; formed by the deposit of crystalline substances excreted in urine; 90% are calcium, 5-8% uric acid, 1-3% cystine.

— Commoner in men than women; occur predominately between ages of 30-60.

— **Treatment goals** are to relieve obstruction, to control infection, to prevent occurrences, and to preserve renal function.

— **Nursing responsibilities** focus primarily on relieving the acute pain and teaching patient/family measures to help prevent recurrent stone formation.

### Specific Considerations, Potential Patient Outcomes, and Nursing Actions:

1) Pain    The patient will experience relief from pain; will perform measures to aid in pain reduction:
— know that pain from a kidney stone is one of the most excruciating pains a pt. can experience; it may radiate to groin & genital areas & be colicky in nature; pts. often say they "can't stand it"; when renal colic occurs, give pain med. stat;
— for dysuria (painful voiding), place pt. in a warm bath X 10 mins.; moist heat to flank area may provide some relief;
— explain cause of pain to pt. (stone moving down the urinary tract); stay with pt. & give emotional support until pain eases;
— when colicky pain subsides, have pt. walk at least 10 mins. Q2H during waking hours (helps stones move downward); if pt. on bed rest, provide active ROM exercises at least TID; see NCPG #1:47.

2) Fluids and Urinary Elimination    The patient will drink at least 2500 cc daily; the patient (or nurse, if patient unable) will measure and strain all urine:
— strain all urine through fine mesh gauze (to detect stones that have passed spontaneously); crush clots & inspect sides of bedpan/urinal for clinging stones; measure urine accurately (to verify patency or blockage of urinary tract); complete

anuria may be due to lodgement of stone in ureter; if no urine in a 4-8 hour period, notify Dr. stat;
— ensure a fluid intake of 2500-3000cc/daily, unless contraindicated; include a quart of cranberry juice in oral fluids (helps acidify urine, thus preventing stone formation); if pt. unable to tolerate oral fluids, an IV may be started;
— inspect urine for degree of hematuria, pus, & concentration; chart findings; monitor urinalysis results & share findings with pt.;
— send all stones/particles to lab.

3) Surgical Intervention

The patient will be prepared for surgery and will recover free of preventable complications:
— if stone does not pass spontaneously, and/or completely suppresses urinary flow, surgery to remove it is indicated; the position of the stone indicates the type of surgery:
  • nephrotomy . . .          simple incision into kidney
  • pyelotomy or
    pyelolithotomy . . .      simple incision into kidney pelvis
  • uretomy . . .             simple incision into ureter
  • cystotomy . . .           simple incision into bladder
  • litholapoxy . . .         instrument inserted through urethra into bladder
— see NCPG #2:44, "General Pre-Op Care," & #2:41, 42, 43, "General Post-Op Care";
— pt. may have nephrostomy tube & a catheter directly into kidney; irrigate only as Dr. orders; carry out strict aseptic technique;
— if pt. had uretomy, expect the abdominal incision to drain urine for nearly 3 weeks; change dressings frequently as wet ones will lead to skin breakdown; provide protective ointments on surrounding skin; irrigate ureteral catheter strictly as ordered, using strict aseptic technique;
— observe for bladder distention, acute retention, signs of hemorrhage; if catheter in bladder, irrigate as ordered, using strict aseptic technique; see NCPG #2:39, "Urethral Catheters";
— when turning & re-positioning pt., ensure that tubes & catheters are not kinked or blocked.

4) Prevention of Stone Formation and Complications

The patient will adhere to a regimen designed to retard stone formation and prevent infection:
— teach pt. about diet restrictions (pt. usually placed on special diet after stone composition has been identified) & role of adequate daily fluid intake (prevents dehydration which leads to stone formation, & dilutes urinary solutes); most pts. are willing to comply in an effort to avoid acute pain & surgery; assess pt.'s knowledge in these areas & teach PRN;

— ensure that pt. knows early signs of urinary tract infection (dull back or flank pain, dysuria, hematuria, frequency) & that infections & calculi often go hand in hand;

— instruct pt. to maintain moderate exercise (as an aid to passage of stones & prevention of stasis of urine) but to avoid very strenuous exercise (as it leads to dehydration); tell pt. to avoid long periods of immobility (leads to venous stasis & infection).

## Discharge Planning and Teaching Objectives/Outcomes

1) (Patient/Family/Significant Other) Knows that calculi may recur and that the best defense is prevention via maintenance of a high fluid intake, avoidance of infection, and adherence to dietary regimen. Knows that dehydration is a significant cause of calculi and to avoid it, as well as strenuous exercise that causes excessive sweating and temporary periods of dehydration.

2) Knows composition of the calculi; has accepted and can follow prescribed dietary regimen; knows to avoid excessive ingestion of minerals & vitamins, especially D.

3) Knows the signs of early urinary tract infection and has resources for early treatment.

**Recommended References**

"Catheters: Indwelling Urethral." NCP Guide #2:39, 2nd Ed., Nurseco, 1980.

"General Postoperative Care." NCP Guides #2:41, 42, 43, 2nd Ed., Nurseco, 1980.

"General Preoperative Care." NCP Guide #2:44, 2nd Ed., Nurseco, 1980.

"How to Break the Kidney Stone Cycle," by Patricia L. Gault. *Nursing 78*, December 1978:24–31.

"Range of Motion Exercises." NCP Guide #1:47, 2nd Ed., Nurseco, 1980.

# The Patient with a Thyroidectomy

**LONG TERM GOAL:**   The patient will resume usual roles at home/work, maintaining adequate rest, nutrition, and emotional stability.

**General Considerations:**
— Surgery is usually done for hyperthyroidism (most common), goiter, or tumor. Tumors are usually benign (called adenomas); malignant tumors are uncommon.
— **Characteristic signs and symptoms** of hyperthyroidism or excessive thyroid hormone are nervousness, emotional hyperexcitability, irritability, rapid pulse, palpitations, flushed skin, fine tremor of hands, increased appetite and weight gain, bugging eyes, elevated BMR, and an increase in PBI.
— Hyperthyroidism frequently appears after an emotional upset or infection, and is more common in women than in men.
— Subtotal thyroidectomy is removal of ⅚ of thyroid tissue; remaining tissue is all that is necessary for normal functioning. Patient is usually on antithyroid drugs pre-op to bring thyroid gland to normal activity.
— **Nursing responsibilities** include preparing patient for surgery and monitoring patient post-op for early signs and symptoms of complications.

**Specific Considerations, Potential Patient Outcomes, and Nursing Actions:**

1) Pre-Op Preparation   The patient will experience no more than a moderate amount of anxiety, hyperexcitability, nervousness, or irritability; will ingest a high-calorie, high protein-CHO diet:
— review NCPG #2:44, "General Pre-Op Care";
— place pt. in a quiet environment, away from seriously ill pts. & any other situations that may serve to increase pt.'s anxiety, nervousness, etc.; control visitors who might disturb pt.; provide quiet music, back rubs & other soothing, calming measures;
— ensure a nutritional intake of a 4-5000 calorie diet daily, high in protein & carbohydrates; know that pt. might be embarrassed by large appetite so provide extra snacks, second helpings, etc., without being asked (diet is needed due to increased metabolic activity and rapid depletion of glycogen reserves).

2) Post-Op Observations   The patient will be monitored closely for detection of early signs of complications; will be free of preventable complications:
— review NCPGs #2:41, 42, 43, "General Post-Op Care";
— inspect dressing for *hemorrhage*, remembering to look at sides & back of neck; icebags may be used over dressing to

help control bleeding & swelling; check with pt. frequently for sensations of pressure or fullness at incision site;

— ask pt. to use voice Q2-4H; note *tone and changes;* voice usually hoarse due to trauma to recurrent laryngeal nerve;

— observe for signs *of cyanosis, noisy breathing* due to trauma per above, or edema of glottis; loosen dressing; keep tracheotomy tray at bedside;

— observe for symptoms of *tetany* (numbness or spasm of hands/feet; muscular twitching; hyperexcitability of nerves); may be due to injury of parathyroid gland;

— observe for signs of *thyroid crisis or storm* (exaggerated hyperthyroid symptoms; pulse of 140-200/min.; increased respirations & elevated temp.); give $O_2$, hypothermia blanket, icepacks, cool sponge, & meds. as ordered;

— report presence of any of above to surgeon at once.

3) Rest and Comfort

The patient will have head and neck supported and positioned adequately; will experience diminishing pain and discomfort:

— position pt. in semi-Fowler's with head supported by pillows and/or sand bags (this will be most comfortable for pt.); turn side to side Q2H, being sure to support pt.'s head in the process (so there is no tension or sutures);

— place tissues, oral fluids, call lites, etc. within easy reach so pt. will not have to turn head to reach them;

— when pt. is able, teach to support own head with hands during movement;

— provide pain medication as ordered, ensuring an adequate amount of rest for pt.;

— maintain a quiet environment, keeping all talking low and to a minimum.

## Discharge Planning and Teaching Objectives/Outcomes

1) (Patient/Family/Significant Other) Understands reasons for and actions of medications and follow-up visits to Dr.'s office; expresses willingness to comply.

2) Understands reasons for rest, relaxation, and nutrition and is able to plan a routine to include these.

3) Can identify factors in home environment that engender emotional tension, and has some alternatives for altering them.

**Recommended References**

"General Preoperative Care." NCP Guide #2:44, 2nd Ed., Nurseco, 1980.

"General Postoperative Care, Parts A, B, C." NCP Guides #2:41, 42, 43, 2nd Ed., Nurseco, 1980.

"Thyroid Disorders," by Janice C. Hallal. *The American Journal of Nursing,* March 1977:418–431.

# The Patient with a Tracheostomy

**Definition:**   A tracheostomy is an opening into the trachea; the procedure itself is called a tracheotomy.

**LONG TERM GOAL:**   The patient will be free of preventable complications, and resume a normal living pattern as soon as possible; or (for a permanent tracheostomy), the patient will care for own tracheostomy and adjust to prescribed medical regimen.

## General Considerations:

— A tracheostomy may be temporary or permanent, and is always done because of an inadequate upper airway. This may be due to:
  - tumor, foreign bodies, edema, nerve or vocal paralysis;
  - inadequate coughing mechanism;
  - shallow respirations due to unconsciousness or paresis; or
  - poor gas exchange across alveolar capillary membrane as a result of extended cardiac or lung surgery, or severe pulmonary edema.
— **Nursing responsibilities** include maintaining a patent airway, preventing complications, and decreasing patient's anxiety and fear to a minimum.

## Specific Considerations, Potential Patient Outcomes, and Nursing Actions:

1) Respiratory Function

The patient will maintain a patent airway, with a tube free of crusts and secretions; the patient will be adequately ventilated:
— know that secretions will be copious, & may be bloody, immediately post-op; suction PRN to keep tube clear;
— use a vented (or Y-tube) catheter to control amount of suction; moisten catheter in sterile water & insert gently, with vent unoccluded; if you encounter resistance, don't force catheter; rather, withdraw it & reinsert; if resistance continues, check for crust formation on inner cannula, or tube displacement (auscultate pt.'s chest & observe for chest expansion);
— cover vent & withdraw catheter; aspirate for only 15 sec. then let pt. rest 15 sec. (this will prevent hypoxia); repeat as often as necessary; 3-5cc of (sterile) saline inserted into tube immediately before suctioning will help liquefy secretions; after suctioning, place your hand 4-5″ away from tube to check on patency; auscultate pt.'s chest to determine if suctioning was effective; listen for breath sounds bilaterally;
— always use sterile catheters; use each one time & discard; wear sterile gloves, use sterile water;
— provide atmospheric humidification via a tracheal mask or other device (helps liquefy secretions, prevent crust formation & tracheitis);
— ensure a fluid intake of 2000cc. daily, unless contraindicated; check with Dr.;

— position pt. in semi-Fowler's or sitting position, to aid breathing & promote comfort;

— chart amount & character of secretions, pt.'s response to procedure, & auscultation findings.

2) Prevention of Complications
The patient will be free of preventable complications such as crust formation, expelled tube, infection:

— use disposable sterile catheters & sterile solutions for suctioning; wear gloves & mask to prevent organisms from being inhaled by pt.;

— remove inner cannula for cleansing when crusts have formed on it; soak cannula in a 3% $H_2O_2$ solution for several minutes; clean with pipe cleaner, rinse with sterile water; let soak in new sterile water for a few minutes before replacing (to ensure no irritating cleaning solutions are left on it); suction outer cannula before replacing inner one; cleaning may need to be done Q1-2H;

— change gauze under tube PRN (never use cotton-filled gauze); change tapes as they become soiled, being sure you have another person with you to hold tube in placing during procedure;

— keep obturator & a Kelly clamp taped to head of bed for stat use if tube should come out;

— deflate cuff periodically to prevent damage to trachea; check with Dr.; review hospital procedure;

— check around tube for bleeding; listen for noisy, obstructed respirations;

— when taking food/fluids, teach pt. to flex head with chin down before swallowing (this narrows the airway & opens the esophagus; when chin is up, airway is fully open).

3) Anxiety
The patient will control his anxiety, keeping it at a minimum level:

— assess what pt. wants and needs to know re: tracheotomy; know that giving information is an effective way to reduce anxiety;

— share with pt. positive signs of adequate breathing, eg. skin color, auscultation findings, blood gas results;

— provide pad & pencil for communication; ensure that pt. has a call bell or some definite way to call for help;

— as soon as pt. able, teach to suction self (this is pt.'s best defense against fear of asphyxia).

4) Decannulation and Discharge Planning
The patient will resume normal breathing pattern without tracheostomy; the patient will suction, clean, and care for own tracheotomy tube:

— when pt. to be weaned from tracheotomy, obstruct tube with a partial plug for 15 minutes; observe for tolerance; remove if any signs of respiratory difficulty; gradually increase size of plug & length of time; pt. should tolerate complete obstruction

of tube with no respiratory difficulty for at least 24 hrs. before removal; if cork is used for a plug, inspect to see that no particles of it have been aspirated;
— if pt. will go home with tube in place, ensure that s/he knows how to clean inner tube, how to proceed if outer tube should become displaced;
— teach pt. to avoid showers, swimming, and other situations when water may get into tube;
— provide a porous covering for tube opening (to screen out dust, etc.); ensure covering does not contain cotton fluff that could be inhaled.

## Discharge Planning and Teaching Objectives/Outcomes
1) (Patient/Family/Significant Other) Knows how to suction tube, remove, clean and replace inner cannula.
2) Knows to avoid and/or take caution with environmental factors that may lead to aspiration of foreign particles, e.g. swimming, showers, dust, wind.

### Recommended References
"Disposable Suction Catheters," by Penny O'Malley and Mary Ann Zankofski. *Nursing '79,* May 1979:71–75.
"Honing Your Respiratory Assessment Technique," by Nancy A. Blackburn and Deborah L. Cebenka. *RN,* May 1980:28–33.
"How to Change Tracheotomy Ties—Easily and Safely," by Bridget O'Donnell and Bennie Gilmore. *Nursing '78,* March 1978:66–69.
"Preventing and Correcting Tube and Cuff Problems in Artificial Airways." *Nursing '80,* January 1980:65–67.

# The Aged Patient: Common Behaviors

**Definition:** Aged—that period of adult development that occurs in the later years of an individual's life cycle. Presently, age 60 is used as a dividing line.

**LONG TERM GOAL:** The individual will accept those physical, emotional, and behavioral changes that occur in the later adult years; will accept support and assistance for maintenance of a sense of self-identity and self-esteem.

## General Considerations:

— Geriatric Nursing Standard #2 (ANA): "In the practice of geriatric nursing, the nurse differentiates between pathological social behavior and the usual life style of each aged individual."

— **Usual Desires/Feelings/Behaviors** include:

1) A desire to *leave a legacy,* something of themselves when they die often becomes a need at this time. It provides a sense of continuity, gives the person a feeling of being able to participate in another's life, even after death.

2) A desire to share *accumulated knowledge and experience* with the young. It may take the form of teaching, counseling, guiding, or sponsoring those who are younger.

3) *An attachment to familiar objects* creates increasing emotional investment in those objects which provide a sense of continuity, comfort, security, satisfaction and which reinforce memories. Examples are: homes, pets, heirlooms, photo albums, old letters, scrapbooks. See "Hoarding Behavior," #9 under Specific Considerations below.

4) *A sense of the life cycle* involves a personal sense of the entire life cycle with an historical perspective and a capacity to summarize and comment upon one's own life. There is a need and value to reminiscing with others; reminiscing is known to be present in those who are the most cheerful and best adapted to reality of present surroundings.

5) *A change in the sense of time* creates a sense of immediacy (less time left), and a need to focus on here and now. Elemental things of life (plants, children) often assume greater significance or value.

— **Common Coping Mechanisms** (the way the person deals with the emotions). It is often advisable to allow the patient to cope in his usual style, since attempts to eliminate one adaptive behavior may result in the substitution of another less satisfactory one.

1) *Denial:* refusal to accept that old age is coming, as is death. It may serve to conserve strength and maintain involvement in activities and others; should not continue to the detriment of health or bring about an earlier death.

2) *Projection:* putting own feelings onto another person or thing; often includes feelings of suspicion about the motivations of others. This paranoid behavior must be clearly distinguished from legitimate complaints.

3) *Fixation:* the inability to move with changes in needs, patterns of living, i.e. refusal to accept the need for outside help or advice as physical strength decreases.
4) *Selective memory:* attempts to tune out or turn away from the painfulness of the present and dwell on the more satisfying past.
5) *Selective sensory reception:* the exclusion of certain stimuli; includes the blocking off of the sensorium that the person feels unprepared to face. This allows the person to maintain some control with regard to the amount of input with which s/he will deal.
6) *Exploitation of age and disability:* use of the changes occurring as a result of aging to obtain secondary gains; can result in freedom from social expectation and often allows the person to try a new identity or a new way of relating; also can cause problems of manipulation and hypochondriacal behavior.
7) *Use of activity or business:* keeping self busy working to keep mind off other matters, warding off unwanted feelings. This is one form of compensation and sublimation.
8) *Insight:* an inner sense of one's self and one's motivations as well as an inner knowledge of the human life cycle; allows the person to make choices about what to oppose, accept, when to struggle and when to acquiesce; includes the willingness and ability to substitute available satisfactions for losses that have occurred.
— **Helpful Nurse/Patient Relationships include:**
  • a listening post for airing feelings, attitudes, beliefs;
  • human warmth, intimacy and use of touch to convey concern, sympathy and love;
  • a feeling of physical and psychological security and comfort;
  • opportunity for mutual growth in maturity, understanding and respect; and
  • emotional-spiritual consolation and counseling.
— The following common emotional reactions and coping mechanisms are discussed in order to show that the older adult has special problems and ways of dealing with them. Be aware that these reactions and adaptive mechanisms *may* be a *normal response* for the situation the person encounters; thus, *assessment* of appropriateness or reality *is crucial.*

**Specific Considerations, Potential Patient Outcomes, and Nursing Actions:**

1) Grief (the result of an actual or anticipated loss)

The patient will accept the process of grieving as normal:
— reassure the pt. that the sadness, anger, loneliness associated with the grief is normal, expected & generally temporary (this information can be extremely helpful to the pt.); when the grief runs its course, the person will be able to look towards the future, make new friends, & make plans about how life will go on;
— see NCPG #1:30, "Responses to Loss . . ."

2) Guilt (the reaction of blaming oneself for omissions & commissions that have occurred; includes the guilt some feel at having outlived friends, family)

The patient will express feelings of guilt and accept support of others to resolve the guilt;
— communicate to the pt. that you respect him, & do not blame him for any shortcomings;
— support attempts at dealing with the guilt; do not give any reassurance about the blaming since this response often evokes anger in the person who feels the guilt.

3) Loneliness (the fear of emotional isolation, of being unable to obtain the warmth and comfort from others that is needed; often occurs as a result of having no one to relate to)

The patient will accept being alone but will also accept input & support of others;
— provide frequent contacts (staff, other pts., visitors) that are expressions of interest, concern & involvement; seek out other pts. with similar interests;
— do not isolate pt.; involve him in planned social groups (friendly club, sports fan club, resocialization and recreational groups).

| | |
|---|---|
| 4) Hopelessness and Depression (an overextended sadness related to a loss and/or aggression (anger) turned inward; occurs in increasing degree & frequency with the older adult) | The patient will feel acceptance and worth and will resolve the loss; will mobilize hope and interest outside self:<br>— signs include insomnia, despair, lethargy, anorexia, loss of interest, somatic complaints, refusal to participate in ADL, sighing heavily;<br>— see NCPG #1:26, "The Patient Experiencing Depression";<br>— refrain from pity, over-concern & rewarding pt. for behaviors such as clinging, whining, self-preoccupation; praise for all efforts at participating in daily care, talking to others, etc. |
| 5) Anxiety (extreme feelings of stress, that things are going to go wrong) | The patient will feel control over his self and parts of his environment:<br>— know that the person becomes concerned with his own life—becoming poor, very sick, and dying soon; anxiety manifests itself in forms of rigid thinking to the exclusion of external stimuli; if someone is extremely anxious, it is important to make as few demands as possible on him; face-to-face contact & conversation with the pt., especially when the focus is his concern, is often helpful in reducing the anxiety;<br>— see NCPG #1:22, "The Patient Experiencing Anxiety";<br>— provide physical activity (walking, needlepoint, knitting, etc.) as a tensional outlet;<br>— use music therapy & dancing for relaxation of tension. |

6) Sense of Impotence & Helplessness (a feeling of lack of power & influence; occurs generally in the older, white, male adult)

The patient will maintain a sense of self-respect by use of choice, control and acceptance of responsibilities:
— give the pt. some control over planning & carrying out his care; let him make as many decisions as possible;
— find some useful, appropriate daily activity & responsibility for pt. to assume (messenger service, dining room duties, help with other pt., janitorial chores, etc.); praise him for efforts & successes.

7) Rage (angry, hostile feelings at the forces attempting to take control of his life; often directed at the indignities, neglect & lack of respect for the older adult)

The patient will express anger appropriately, and to the person with whom s/he is angry:
— this reaction is necessary & important, especially to the resolution of the grief process;
— allow pt. to express these feelings without reprimands;
— physically destructive rage should be dealt with by use of limit-setting; praise of constructive or verbally expressed feelings is necessary in order to prevent destructive rate;
— refer to NCPG's #1:20, #1:21, "The Patient Manifesting Aggression," "The Patient Manifesting Anger."

8) Hypochon-driasis (overconcern with the body processes, illness, somatic complaints)

The patient will focus on activities and interactions with others:
— show a sincere interest & desire to assess accurately & realistically all complaints, but refrain from showing excessive sympathy or concern;
— do not acknowledge the same complaints over & over by giving pt. your attention to them; rather, give pt. attention for positive efforts, e.g. doing own ADL, participating in activities, etc.
— do not ask pt. how s/he feels periodically, but base your evaluation & intervention on observed behavior & objective signs;
— keep pt. busily involved in purposeful social or occupational activities & conversation outside himself.

| 9) Hoarding (saving food, string, paper sacks, envelopes, & misc. items) | The patient will surround self with familiar items of sentimental & personal value, will meet environmentally–safe, clean standards for daily living; |

- provide reasonable shelves, closet & drawer space for photos, clocks, plants, letters, books, & cosmetic articles;
- explain & enforce (kindly and firmly) rules for securing money, expensive jewelry, other valuables; provide pt./family with detailed list of items taken;
- clean the pt.'s unit & bedside stand with his permission & presence;
- try to obtain pt. & family's cooperation re: storage of perishable food; explain that it attracts insects, rodents;
- provide pts. with time alone to sort, look through & re-pack various personal items, mementoes, etc. into suitcase or private box; show pt. where these will be kept;
- have bulletin boards or spaces to hang greeting cards, grandchildren's art work, etc.

**Recommended References**

*Aging and Mental Health* by R. Butler & M. Lewis. St. Louis: The C.V. Mosby Co., 1973.
"Breaking Through the Cobwebs of Confusion in the Elderly," by Carolyn Stevens. *Nursing '74*, August 1974.
"Finding and Using Your Patient's Strengths." Nursing Grand Rounds. *Nursing '79*, March 1979:40–45.
"Recognizing and Reducing Emotional Problems in the Aged," by Irene Burnside. *Nursing '77*, March 1977:56–59.
"Responses to Loss: the Grief and Mourning Process," NCP Guide #1:31, 2nd Ed., Nurseco, 1980.
"Standards for Geriatric Nursing Practice" by ANA Division on Geriatric Nursing. *American Journal of Nursing*, September 1970:1894–1897.
"Supporting the Hospitalized Elderly Person," by Ann Lore, *American Journal of Nursing*, March 1979:496–499.
"The Aged Patient: Physiology of Aging." NCP Guide #2:33, 2nd Ed., Nurseco, 1980.
"The Aged Patient: Transition to Communal Living." NCP Guide #2:27, 2nd Ed., Nurseco, 1980.
"The Patient Displaying Manipulation." NCP Guide #1:29, 2nd Ed., Nurseco, 1980.
"The Patient Experiencing Anxiety." NCP Guide #1:22, 2nd Ed., Nurseco, 1980.
"The Patient Experiencing Confusion." NCP Guide #1:23, 2nd Ed., Nurseco, 1980.
"The Patient Experiencing Depression." NCP Guide #1:26, 2nd Ed., Nurseco, 1980.
"The Patient Manifesting Aggression." NCP Guide #1:20, 2nd Ed., Nurseco, 1980.
"The Patient Manifesting Anger." NCP Guide #1:21, 2nd Ed., Nurseco, 1980.
"The Staff Called Mrs. Jepson's Care Plan 'Resocialization,' I Called it a Repressive Regimen," by Joan Schuettler. *Nursing '74*, August 1974:10–12.

# The Aged Patient: Transition to Communal Living

**Definition:** Communal living is that situation in which the older person changes his mode of living from the usual (family or living alone) to that of living in the same environment with others, e.g. board and care homes, extended care facilities.

**LONG TERM GOAL:** The patient will have an environment and life style that satisfies his need for self-esteem, independence, familiarity, and adaptation.

## General Considerations:
— Geriatric Nursing Standard #7 (ANA): "The nurse employs a variety of methods to promote effective communication and social interaction of aged persons with individuals, family and other groups."
— Geriatric Nursing Standard #8 (ANA): "The nurse together with the older person designs, changes or adapts the physical and psychosocial environment to meet his needs within the limitations imposed by the situation."
— **Health and economics** are the major influences affecting the individual's movement to a communal lifestyle.
— For many older adults, aging represents less interest in social involvement but an **increased** *interest in unstructured, solitary* activities.
— **Maintenance** *of self-esteem* is a necessary prerequisite to adaptation to the aging process and/or communal living.
— **Nursing responsibilities** include maintaining an adult relationship with the patient even when certain patient needs are similar to those of a child, and focusing on the advocacy of the older adult's need to maintain his usual habits as much as possible.

## Specific Considerations, Potential Patient Outcomes, and Nursing Actions:

1) Maintenance of Individual Identity

The patient will live in an environment conducive to adaptation, individual needs, and functioning and will develop a daily routine that maintains independence:
— assess personal needs with pt. (& family when needed & desired) on admission; include the following:
  • amount, type & conditions for privacy;
  • desire & need for social contact with others;
  • usual pattern of ADL, e.g. bathing, elimination, sleeping routines;
  • usual habits, hobbies, need for telephone, religious involvement;
  • amount of independence & dependence, e.g. What things can patient do alone? What things does s/he need assistance with?
  • medications used;
  • maintenance of relationship with family via visits, calls, letters, etc.;
— orient pt. & family to home & grounds; point out facilities; introduce to other pts.; explain that staff will adapt the facility &

pt's. routines to each other as much as possible;
— encourage & allow pt. to retain & use as many personal belongings (including clothing) as s/he wishes;
— allow pt. to replace standard furnishings with personal ones; e.g. pillow, clock, bedspread, pictures, clothes, etc., in order to maintain contact with reality & link this new environment to that of his usual home;
— facilitate interest & participation in occupational therapy, hobbies, crafts, social groups, etc., but give pt. a chance to be alone as well.

2) Restoration to Adaptive Coping

The patient will deal with the loss of usual style of living and accommodate to communal living:
— identify & discuss with pt. those aspects of the transition to communal living that are most fearsome or threatening to him, e.g. loneliness, dependence, abandonment;
— permit pt. to respond behaviorally to the loss in *any* non-destructive way (see NCPG #1:31, "Responses to Loss");
— identify any *other losses* the pt. may be responding to, i.e. loss of body part or body part functioning;
— identify & point out to the pt. those areas that are not lost & are significant to his adaptation, e.g. family, friends, old memories, mementos, etc.
— plan & evaluate the nursing care *with* the pt.; allow him to make as many decisions as possible (taking away all power or choices can produce dependency, resentment, fear, distrust);
— plan time & opportunity for the pt. to meet his social needs, i.e. time for friends & family to visit, privacy for meeting sexual needs, time & opportunity to play cards, shuffleboard, bingo, etc.; often these needs supersede physical needs & nursing judgment requires reviewing each case individually rather than maintaining a set pattern;
— allow pt. to decide about availability & use of clocks, calendars, TV, radio, etc.

**Recommended References**

"Autonomy: A Continuing Developmental Task," by Shirley Dresen. *American Journal of Nursing*, August 1978:1344–1346.
"Caring for the Aged." *American Journal of Nursing*, December 1973:2049–2066 (a series of 5 articles).
"Caring for the Elderly," by Joan E. Bowers. *Nursing '78*, January, 1978:42–47.
"Considerate Care of the Elderly: Little Things Mean a Lot," by J. Cahall and D. Smith. *Nursing '75*, September 1975:38–40.
"Geriatric Care: Let's Make It More Than Physical Care," by Sister Michael Sibille. *Nursing '75*, July 1975:54–55.
"How Do the Elderly View Their World," by Mildred Hogstel. *American Journal of Nursing*, August 1978:1335–1336.
"Pace: An Approach to Improving the Care of the Elderly," by Faye Abdellah et al. *American Journal of Nursing*, June 1979:1109–1110.
"Standards for Geriatric Nursing Practice," by ANA Division on Geriatric Nursing. *American Journal of Nursing*, September 1970:1894–1897.
"Responses to Loss: the Grief and Mourning Process," NCP Guide #1:31, 2nd Ed., Nurseco, 1980.
"The Aged Patient: Common Behaviors," NCP Guide #2:26, 2nd Ed., Nurseco, 1980.
*The Psychosocial Needs of the Aged: Selected Papers.* The Publications Office, Ethel Percy Andrus Gerontology Center, University of Southern California, Los Angeles: 1973.

# The Burn Patient: Common Behaviors

**LONG TERM GOAL:**   The patient will recover from the burn physically and emotionally; the patient will resolve the loss it created and make future plans and goals involving creative and economic activities.

## General Considerations:
— Any burn, including a sunburn, is a discomfort, but 2nd or 3rd degree burns can be considered a physical and emotional trauma.
— **A burn establishes** a temporary or permanent loss of body function, possibly a body part, self-image, and usual roles.
— **Responses to the loss** may include the following fears: disfigurement, physical discomfort, death, mutilation, abandonment, surgical procedures, long convalescence. Many of these fears may be real, and resolution may take several weeks based on the course of treatment and the individual's response to it. Routine answers of "everything will be fine" should not be given to the burn patient.
— **A serious burn will cause prolonged** separation from significant others and community involvement. This separation may result in feelings of inadequacy and rejection on the part of the patient as well as the arousal of dependency conflicts. A common feeling is that of guilt, manifested by reliving the accident, attempting to resolve why it occurred, and sometimes blaming self or others for it. These patients often associate the pain they are feeling with punishment, i.e. the pain is punishment for their causing or not doing enough to prevent the present outcome of the accident.
— **Some common behavioral responses** are denial, delusion/illusion, resignation, rationalization, suppression of feelings; often unexpressed feelings and emotional needs will result in increased somatic complaints.
— The burn patient is in an emotionally hazardous situation, which may or may not turn into a crisis; see NCPG #2:31 #2:35, "Crisis Intervention."

## Specific Considerations, Potential Patient Outcomes, and Nursing Actions:
1) Immediate Response to Recognition of the Losses

The patient will verbally express his anxieties, fears, sadness, and anger associated with loss of function that is a result of the burn:
— pt. & family will go through initial stages of grief & mourning: shock, disbelief, denial (see NCPG #1:31, "Responses to Loss"); allow them to use any of these adaptive defense mechanisms to cope with this current situation/crisis, but do not permit destructive behavior;
— find out the pt.'s usual way of coping with stress (withdrawal? physically/verbally aggressive? talk out conflict? assess situation, then act? act before assessing?); this information is an important indicator of possible pt. behavioral responses to treatment;

— assess importance & impact of appearance changes; discuss impact with pt. & family;
— a burn is a devastating injury; do not push pt. into acceptance or beginning awareness of this devastation before s/he is ready;
— orientation may be interspersed with delirium & confusion; carefully assess all parameters (electrolytes, vital signs, wound appearance) to discern if disorientation is a physical or emotional response; reinforce reality, time of day/day of week/ name of hospital, etc.; if related to a physical cause, pt. may perceive it as a loss, or even fear of going crazy; explain that this is not so, & is temporary;
— realize & share with pt./family that the behavioral responses/feelings they are experiencing are normal, expected & temporary;
— give pt. specific choices to enhance/sustain efforts at independence & to lessen feelings of helplessness (determining times for meals, dressings, etc.); but set limits & do not give pt. choices about type of medical treatment;
— some of the most helpful things a nurse can do for the pt./family in this hazardous situation are to *listen* (provide a calm accepting attitude) and *manipulate the environment* to provide support (move bed, adjust lights, move curtain); see NCPG #2:29, "Body Image Disturbance" and #2:35, "Crisis Intervention";
— plan for frequent meetings with pt.'s family to provide information, reassurance, support & feedback; informing & supporting the family can establish them as supportive to the care of the pt.; recognition of their needs and responses is absolutely necessary to successful interactions;
— consult with a psychiatric nursing specialist or mental health consultant on a continuing basis & PRN.

2) Adaptation to Long Term Treatment & Rehabilitation

The patient will show evidence of involvement in his care by giving direction to his care; where appropriate, patient will use the reassurance, support and input from others to make progress towards self care:
— understand that with the need to deal with losses, long term hospitalization & changes in self-image, most seriously–burned pts. experience personality changes; these changes often occur during & at the end of a cycle of behavioral responses to the changing self-image; this cycle is **denial,** leading to **repression** (unconscious banishment of unacceptable ideas, effect, or impulses), which extends to **suppression,** (the conscious effort to control and conceal unacceptable ideas and thoughts), and finally, **acceptance;**
— know that the personality changes are often greatly affected by pt. experiences of being near death; changes may include a different interpretation of the meaning of life & death, a different, changed attitude toward finances, life style, role, etc., & may cause fears & conflicts to arise between pt. and family;

— assess the extent of these personality changes, considering pre-burn personality & usual coping mechanisms;

— pt. may need support & some introspective assistance in dealing with the pt./family relationship since hospitalization may have necessitated changes in roles among family members; this support should be in the form of listening, exploration of thoughts, feelings & plans with regard to changes in self-image & role of family members (see NCPG #2:29, "Body Image Disturbance"); sitting with pt. at least once a day can help him with this task.

3) Restoration to Adaptive Coping

The patient will accept changes in his body structure and/or function; will be involved with his significant others; will make future life goals and will verbally discuss the changes in life style caused by the burn:

— plan experiences for the pt. where s/he can control the situation & succeed in it; praise pt. for whatever efforts are made;

— encourage pt.'s efforts at physical rehabilitation; generally this process is slow & each step must be rewarded so that there is motivation to continue;

— involve pt. in activities (e.g. creative OT) that provide success & make pt. feel useful & important;

— spend time weekly with pt.'s family to inform them of his progress; praise them for their efforts in coping; support their efforts to work with the pt. to maintain open lines of communication;

— plan for at least a weekly health team conference to discuss pt.'s progress, needs, behavioral interventions, discharge plans;

— plan at least a weekly nursing meeting where staff can openly discuss their own concerns & feelings about caring for severely burned pts.; include discussions of feelings about death, disfigurement, personality changes;

— work on ways of enhancing appearance with the pt. & family since burn injuries can often appear grotesque to the pt. & others.

## Discharge Planning and Teaching Objectives/Outcomes

1) (Patient/Family/Significant Other) Can discuss the impact of returning to home after a prolonged confinement.

2) Can verbally describe the physical and emotional needs necessary to function at home.

3) Has plans for future that are specific and include activities that meet economic, creative, and social needs.

**Recommended References**
"Burns: Breaking the Anger-Despair Cycle," by Nursing Grand Rounds. *Nursing '75* May 1975:44–50.
"Crisis Intervention: Adaptation to General Nursing," NCP Guide #2:35, 2nd Ed., Nurseco, 1980.
"Motivating the Unmotivated Patient," by Mary Anne Kavchak et al. *Nursing '74*, February 1974:31–36.
"Responses to Loss: the Grief and Mourning Process." NCP Guide #1:31, 2nd Ed., Nurseco, 1980.
"Sam, The Patient Nobody Wanted to Visit," by Sharon Warlik. *Nursing '78*, July 1978:56–58.
"Special Behavioral Problems of the Burned Child," by Laura Campbell. *American Journal of Nursing*, February 1976:220–224.
"The Patient Experiencing a Body Image Disturbance." NCP Guide #2:29, 2nd Ed., Nurseco, 1980.
"The Patient Needing Crisis Intervention." NCP Guide #2:31, 2nd Ed., Nurseco, 1980.

# The Patient Experiencing a Body Image Disturbance

**Definition:**  The inability of an individual to perceive and/or adapt to his body, or part of it, in a changed form.

**LONG TERM GOAL:**  The patient will be able to manage his own life, make future goals and live with others while being aware that his body has changed.

## General Considerations:
— **Body image** results from internal development as well as environmental experiences, including input from others, societal views, cultural practices, and previous experiences with persons whose bodies have been changed.
— **Nursing responsibilities** include an awareness of the causes of body image disturbances which are:
(1)  a real or anticipated loss of a body part and/or its usual functioning (colostomy, diabetes);
(2)  neurological disorders resulting in changes in locomotion and posture (e.g. paralysis);
(3)  metabolic or toxic disorders resulting in changes in body structure (e.g. kidney failure);
(4)  progressively-deforming disorders (e.g. arthritis);
(5)  acute dismemberment disorders (e.g. amputation, mastectomy);
(6)  personality development disorders (e.g. schizophrenia).
— **Nursing assessment** involves an awareness of the behavioral manifestations indicative of a body image disturbance and include:
(1)  refusal to continue functioning at any level, to believe any change has occurred and/or to look at altered body part;
(2)  inability to care for self or perform any activities of daily living;
(3)  withdrawal; hostility;
(4)  any behavior indicative of a response to a loss (e.g. shock, denial, anger); see NCPG #1:31, "Responses to Loss . . ."
— **Nursing interventions** should focus on assisting the patient to adapt to the loss which results from change and reinforcing those areas of continued daily functioning.

## Specific Considerations, Potential Patient Outcomes, and Nursing Actions:

1) Immediate Response to Recognition of a Body Image Disturbance

The patient will be able to verbally state that a loss-change in body has occurred:
— provide openings for the pt. to express feelings by validating your observations & feelings with him (e.g. "You look down in the dumps; how are things going for you today?" or "You seem upset/sad. Are you?"); be a good listener & accept what pt. verbalizes; if s/he expresses anger or hostile feelings, remember not to take them personally; s/he may be handling them in the only way possible;

— focus on the pt.'s feelings & deal with the presenting behavior, e.g. if s/he is denying a body change that has actually occurred, do not challenge the pt.;

— determine what the body image change means to the pt.; how does s/he think it will affect his life? If you think his perceptions are unrealistic, do not challenge them at this time; the best intervention you can provide is the opportunity for him to share these perceptions & feelings with you;

— accept any body changes you observe in the pt.; if pt. is repulsed or ashamed of physical changes, s/he will be watching the faces of others for negative signs;

— provide basic needs for pt.; s/he may be very dependent on staff at this time;

— let the pt. know that the feelings & concerns s/he is experiencing are normal & that you are there to listen to him as well as help him cope.

2) Restoration to Adaptive Coping

The patient will accept the body alterations and verbalize how these will affect job, family life, view of life:

— give positive reinforcement for pt.'s efforts to adapt; his behavior will indicate when he starts to accept alterations in his body (may ask questions; will start to look at the incision, dressings, etc.); accept, but do not support expressions of denial;

— if a prosthesis will be used, assist pt. in his choice by providing information & arranging for a visit by someone from Colostomy Club, Reach for Recovery, or other appropriate group; let pt. determine time of visit, but try to arrange it as soon as possible;

— involve pt. in self care activities; begin slowly & add new activities one at a time; reinforce any efforts to participate;

— include in nursing care plan pt.'s perception of what the body change means to him, the objectives & nursing actions prescribed; share plan with all care givers, including family;

— tell others how they can help pt. by listening, supporting reality, allowing expressions of anger, denial, & not challenging them; permitting pt. to cry & giving positive reinforcement for all pt.'s efforts to cope/adapt;

— praise these others for their efforts to help pt.;

— hold a team conference, include family if you wish, & share information on "The Grief and Mourning Process" & "Crisis Intervention" (NCPG's #2:31, 35) with each other; discuss what parts of these concepts apply to this pt. at this time; revise the care plan PRN.

**Discharge Planning and Teaching Objectives/Outcomes**
1) (Patient/Family/Significant Other) Can identify how body has changed.
2) Can verbalize the fact that sadness and other feelings related to the loss are normal and part of the grief and mourning process.
3) Can accept continued support and positive input from significant others.
4) Can utilize community resources such as Reach for Recovery, Colostomy Club, to provide ongoing support, reassurance, and assistance in recovery.

**Recommended References**
"Crisis Intervention: Adaptation to General Nursing." NCP Guide #2:35, 2nd Ed., Nurseco, 1980.
"How To Make The Most of Body Image Theory in Nursing Practice," by Joanne McCloskey. *Nursing '76,* May 1976:68–72.
"Reestablishing Body Image," by Elaine Smith et al. *American Journal of Nursing,* March 1977:445–447.
"Responses to Loss: The Grief and Mourning Process," NCP Guide #1:31, 2nd Ed., Nurseco, 1980.
"Symposium on the Concept of Body Image." *Nursing Clinics of North America,* Philadelphia: W. B. Saunders Company, December 1972:593–707.
"The Patient Needing Crisis Intervention." NCP Guide #2:31, 2nd Ed., Nurseco, 1980.

# The Patient Experiencing the Impact of Another's Cardiac Arrest

**LONG TERM GOAL:**  The patient will be able to verbalize anxiety and fear related to the cardiac arrest of another patient.

**General Considerations:**
— Persons seeing the mobilization and fast action/talk of others may perceive all kinds of occurrences. Information and reassurances as well as the opportunity to talk about the incident will reduce and/or eliminate misperception and physiological stress responses induced by the event.
— **Nursing responsibilities** include an awareness that anxiety or stress is a response to an event and it requires the patient to cope with a new situation. Nurses should know that *isolation* can cause exaggeration of feelings or distortion of reality and is often created by closing doors and/or curtains around the patient, preventing family from visiting, withholding information from patient, and leaving him alone.
— **Nursing assessment** includes observing for behavioral manifestations such as:
  (1)  Acute anxiety/fear that same might happen to him,
  (2)  Any behavior indicative of a reaction to stress/anxiety (e.g. withdrawal, anger, crying, denial, asking questions),
  (3)  Increased physical symptoms.
— **Nursing intervention** should focus on decreasing the fear and anxiety created by the possible loss of life of another patient. The patient needs reassurance, understanding, accurate information and staff realization that his reaction is normal for the situation. Isolating patients without any follow up only causes increased anxiety and physiological stress.

**Specific Considerations, Potential Patient Outcomes, and Nursing Actions:**
1) Immediate Response to Recognition of Anxiety, Fear

The patient will be able to express his fears regarding the event of the other patient and possible loss of his own life:
— at least one nurse should focus on other pts. on the unit who can see/hear efforts being made to resuscitate another pt.;
— do not permit large numbers of professionals to stand around unnecessarily, watching CPR efforts; rather, have these people sit with other pts.;
— allow pt.'s family to stay with him, if they are present;
— share with them that another pt. is going through a crisis & that everything possible is being done;
— if additional family members wish to help by staying with another pt. during this time, let them do so;
— maintain staff visibility for the pt.;
— when necessary to close doors/curtains, give an honest explanation as to the reasons.

2) Restoration
   to Adaptive
   Coping

The patient will be able to verbalize that crisis events cause fear but will be able to talk realistically about the event, possible arrest, and his own illness situation:
— answer all questions the pt. may ask you; do not give false answers or reassurance; outline (when appropriate) what measures are available for emergency treatment to provide quick, immediate action;
— provide any physical needs/care for the pt.;
— be aware that your actions & presence will help reassure pt. that s/he is safe & being cared for; often, just sitting quietly with the pt., sharing this time together, will provide needed support & help pt. get through this crucial period;
— refer to NCPG #1:22, "The Patient Experiencing Anxiety" & #1:28, "The Patient Experiencing Fear";
— administer soporific drugs as ordered & as needed for those pts. who need additional methods to relieve anxiety, etc.;
— after the crisis is past, share the outcome with the other pts., again eliciting their feelings, concerns, reactions; point out positive signs of their progress as you see them (favorable responses in pulse, EKG, lab. reports, etc.).

**Discharge Planning and Teaching Objectives/Outcomes**
1) (Patient/Family/Significant Other) Can ask for situational support during or just after a crisis event involving another in a similar situation.
2) Can separate own feelings and experiences from that of other patients and verbally state the reality of the event.

**Recommended References**
"Helping the Family Cope with a Cardiac Arrest" by Mary Ann Ryan. *Nursing '74*, August 1974:80–81.
"The Patient Experiencing Anxiety." NCP Guide #1:22, 2nd Ed., Nurseco, 1980.
"The Patient Experiencing Fear." NCP Guide #1:28, 2nd Ed., Nurseco, 1980.

# The Patient Needing Crisis Intervention

**Definition:**  Crisis intervention refers to those approaches used to restore a patient to a state of emotional equilibrium from one of disequilibrium (the crisis state).

**LONG TERM GOAL:**  The patient will achieve adaptive resolution of the crisis; will return to his usual job/roles with a realistic perception of what has occurred and with adequate coping mechanisms.

**General Considerations:**
— Read NCPG #2:35, "Crisis Intervention: Adaptation to General Nursing."
— In a non-psychiatric setting, the major loss or hazard is often situational: what brought the patient in, e.g. physical illness, trauma. Additional losses may include: loss of job, of independence, of usual role functioning, of usual living style (as in transfer to a nursing home).
— **Common manifestations** of a crisis include:
  — overwhelming feelings of helplessness, hopelessness
  — feelings of inability to cope anymore
  — feelings of loss of control over own life
  — decreased ability to carry out own activities of daily living
  — increased dependence on others
  — high anxiety; may develop into a panic state
  — inability to work and/or carry out usual roles
  — increased somatic complaints
— **Nursing responsibilities** focus initially on adequate assessment:
  — assessment of the patient and his current situation will tell you if the patient is in an actual crisis or in a hazardous situation. If the former, the objective is to help the patient achieve adaptive resolution of the crisis; if the latter, the objective is to prevent a crisis from occurring.
  — although hazardous situations create stress for *all* people, why do they develop into a crisis for some and not for others? This has to do with the presence or absence of balancing factors; assessment of these factors is essential.

**Specific Considerations, Potential Patient Outcomes, and Nursing Actions:**

1) Immediate
Response to
Recognition of
an Actual or
Potential Crisis

The patient will verbalize what s/he is experiencing; will express a feeling of decreasing anxiety; will identify those components that are most anxiety-producing:
— read NCPG #1:22, "The Patient Experiencing Anxiety";
— ask the pt. what is happening to him right now (scared? afraid? panicky? hopeless?) what occurred to make him feel like this? (accident? new diagnosis? new equipment in room?);
— allow pt. to respond at length & in detail to your questions; do not challenge any statements; try to determine exactly what is *most* threatening to him; listen & encourage pt. to keep talking;
— determine the real/anticipated pt. loss/losses involved; assess behavior in light of the Grief & Mourning Process (see NCP Guide #1:31, "Responses to Loss . . .");
— change the environment to reduce impact of the hazard, e.g. change room, allow family to stay, etc.;
— ask the pt. what you could do to make him feel better right now; if at all possible, provide it;
— provide basic needs; pt. may be very dependent in ADL; allow this dependency to occur for the immediate time;
— when you leave room, tell pt. when you will be back & return when you say you will;
— share information with pt. re: tests, procedures, etc.; tell him what he can expect (will help decrease feelings of anxiety, hopelessness);
— when the pt.'s behavior indicates that s/he is beginning to adapt or cope (begins to ask questions, focus on reality), support & reinforce reality; share with pt. how you see it; ask him to clarify or validate your perceptions.

2) Restoration to
Adaptive
Coping

The patient will express feelings of decreased hopelessness and helplessness; will regain a degree of control over own life; will develop alternate solutions to cope with current problem:
— continue to give pt. as much information as s/he wants to know about hospitalization, treatment, therapy; ask for feedback to ensure pt. understanding;
— help pt. increase independence in ADL: involve in self-care, slowly at first, then gradually adding more activities;
— provide opportunities for pt. to make decisions about daily care (this gives pt. some control over own life); praise pt. for making decisions, for coping with current stress, for helping self to feel better;
— help pt. brainstorm alternate solutions to current problem & look at the pros & cons of each one; don't tell pt. what to do, but ask if one of the solutions could possibly work for him;
— assess pt.'s perceptions of what has happened to him & correct any misperceptions;

- encourage pt. to share feelings, perceptions, new coping options, etc. with family/significant others; encourage them, in turn, to support pt.; explain to all the importance of the three balancing factors in pt. maintenance of equilibrium;
- check the effectiveness of pt.'s new coping options by asking what s/he would do if confronted with a situation similar to the one s/he has just experienced; reinforce positive adaptation & coping & teach PRN.

## Discharge Planning and Teaching Objectives/Outcomes

1) (Patient/Family/Significant Other) Has a realistic expectation of what occurred and can verbalize what patient was feeling at the time.
2) Has adequate situational supports in the form of family, friends, job.
3) Can verbalize at least three options s/he can use to cope with stress.
4) Has name of a community resource to go to if s/he finds self in another hazardous situation with which s/he cannot cope.

**Recommended References**

"Crisis Intervention: Adaptation to General Nursing." NCP Guide #2:35, 2nd Ed., Nurseco, 1980.

"Crisis Intervention in Acute Care Areas," by Sandra H. Huenzi and Mary V. Fenton, *American Journal of Nursing*, May 1975:830–834.

"Responses to Loss: the Grief and Mourning Process." NCP Guide #1:31, 2nd Ed., Nurseco, 1980.

"Symposium on Crisis Intervention," *Nursing Clinics of North America*, Philadelphia: W.B. Saunders Company, March 1974:1–96.

# The Aged Patient: Exercises for Patients Over 65

**GOALS:**  The patient's circulation and oxygenation of all body tissues will be improved; the patient will express reduced muscular aches and stiffness and will experience relaxation of mind and body; the patient will be more flexible and mobile with fewer complications of impaired mobility.

### General Considerations:
— Medical authorization to participate in the following exercises should be obtained in writing for each patient.
— Exercising should be fun, feel good and help to meet the above goals. They should be done regularly, i.e. at least three times a week, preferably once a day.
— **Remember:** strength and endurance are *not* the goals of exercise for elderly persons; patients should start slowly and do each exercise only once or twice; they should rest nearly a minute between different exercises.
— see NCPG #1:47, "Range of Motion Exercises," for patients confined to bed or unable to be up in a chair for at least 45 minutes.
— See recommended references for standing exercises to use with ambulatory elderly persons who are alert and more able than chairbound, convalescing and/or senile patients for whom these exercises below are designed.

### Suggested Format:
— Assemble patients in semi-circle groups of 5 to 10, all sitting comfortably and securely in armchairs or locked wheelchairs with feet resting on floor. Provide each patient with a hand towel.
— Have an assistant to help you observe tolerance limits of patients, to show patients how to perform exercises correctly within individual abilities, to provide suitable room ventilation without drafts, to arrange for pleasant, rhythmic music accompaniment, and to serve nourishing liquids after exercise period.
— While seated, facing patients, demonstrate each exercise slowly, then help patients to do the exercise once the first day and then two or three times on successive days as tolerated.

### Specific Exercises:
1) Breathing & Blowing:   Take 3 to 5 long, slow, deep breaths, holding each for at least three seconds, then exhaling slowly, blowing outward.

2) Funny Faces:   (a) Open eyes wide; open mouth wide, stick out tongue as far as possible, then return face to normal facial position.
(b) Wrinkle face like a prune; relax, then smile broadly.

3) Head Rolling:   Stretch neck, bending head forward to touch chin to chest; then tilt head to side, rolling it slowly backward; pause, then tilt head to opposite side, finishing with head bent forward again to rest. Repeat to opposite direction.

4) Shoulder Shrugging:   Clasp hands in front of chest; lift shoulders up in a shrug, then return to normal position; lift right shoulder only, lower it; then lift left shoulder only, lower and relax.

5) Wing Flapping:   Bend elbows, tucking hands in armpits; wave bent arms up and down as if flying. Straighten arms outward, holding them at shoulder level and make 5 small circles with the arms forward, then backward.

6) Swim Strokes:   Extending arms forward, reach and pull each arm alternately in the standard swim stroke.

7) Surrender Wave:   Holding handtowel in both hands, reach arms overhead and wave arms, as if to surrender or to attract help.

8) Fist & Finger Flexion:   Resting arms in lap, make a tight fist with each hand; then open hands and fingers widely spreading them apart; turn palms upward, then palms downward.

9) Wrist & Hand Circles:   Holding hands in a relaxed position, flop them up and down; then make circles, as if turning an egg beater or stirring a batter.

10) Rag Doll Trunk Slump:   With feet flat on floor, arms resting in lap, straighten trunk, holding head erect; take a breath, then slump for a moment like a rag doll; straighten up again.

11) Knee Spread:   Open legs wide, spreading bent knees and legs apart as far as comfortable; relax, then return legs to normal sitting position, holding knees and legs tightly together for a moment; then relaxing again.

12) Leg Lift:   Place hand towel under knee, holding ends in each hand; lift knee upward as far as possible while sitting; then lower leg and rest; repeat with opposite knee.

13) Feet & Ankle Circles:   Lifting one foot off floor, circle it in either direction; then lift other foot off floor and circle it; then lift both feet off floor and circle them simultaneously.

14) Toe Wiggle:   With slippers off, wiggle toes; curl and straighten.

15) Clapping:   Applaud yourselves, keeping time together.

**Recommended References**

"Exercises for the Elderly," by Dr. Herman L. Kamenetz. Armour Pharmaceutical Company, (P.O. Box 1022, Chicago, IL 60690).

"Exercises to Help the Elderly—to Live Longer, Stay Healthier and Be Happier," by Lawrence J. Frankel and Betty Byrd Richard. *Nursing 77*, December 1977:58–63.

"Range of Motion Exercises," NCP Guide #1:47, 2nd Ed., Nurseco, 1980.

# The Aged Patient: Physiology of Aging

**LONG TERM GOAL:** The patient will verbally acknowledge the physiological changes that normally accompany the aging process; the patient will maintain an optimum level of health consistent with limitations of the aging process.

**General Considerations:**
— Geriatric Nursing Standard #1 (ANA): The nurse observes and interprets minimal as well as gross signs and symptoms associated with both normal aging and pathologic changes and institutes appropriate nursing measures."
— Geriatric Nursing Standard #5 (ANA): "The nurse supports and promotes normal physiologic functioning of the older person."
— As an individual ages, s/he has a decreased capacity to coordinate activities of many body systems and to adjust to change. Basically, the body slows down and reserve capacities are diminished. **The responsibility of the nurse** is to know the physiology of aging, and to help the aged individual maintain homeostasis, adapt to and accept the changes occurring in his body systems.
— **Common physiological changes** occurring in the older adult include:

**Systems & Changes**
1) **Cardiovascular:**
   — diminished cardiac reserve;
   — elastic fibers in blood vessels progressively straighten, split and fragment;
   — thickening and loss of elasticity of valves;
   — increase in fat deposits around heart;
   — decrease in cardiac output and stroke volume;
   — pulse reacts slowly to changes or stress and takes longer to return to normal;
   — blood vessel walls become thicker, harder, less elastic, resulting in slower circulation, "small" strokes, poorer vision, slower healing, slower adjustment to skin temperature changes, etc.

**Implications for Nursing**
1) **Cardiovascular:**
   — take vital signs only after patient has rested (in order to insure accurate, non-stress related reading);
   — examine peripheral circulation periodically: check for cold extremities, decreased peripheral pulse rates; provide comfort measures consistent with these changes: extra blankets, flannel sheet blankets, etc.;
   — allow time for rest between activities; provide limited-exertion activities; assist patient with activities of daily living PRN;
   — give good foot care; see NCPG #1:39, "Care of the Feet";
   — listen to apical pulse in various cardiac auscultation sites to assess cardiac changes.

2) **Respiratory:**
   — the lungs are more rigid, resulting in reduced capacity to cough and deep breathe, increasing the chances of complications in response to immobility;
   — because elastin fibers become thicker, aggregate and less elastic, the muscles of ribs and chest are more rigid and breathing becomes less efficient;
   — arteriosclerotic changes in blood vessels cause a decrease in the $O_2$ and $CO_2$ exchange and $O_2$ use.

3) **Gastrointestinal:**
   — decreased secretion of enzymes; indigestion common;
   — decreased absorption of nutrients and minerals;
   — reduced motility of stomach;
   — slowing of peristalsis;
   — decrease in sense of smell and taste;
   — additional problems caused by problems with teeth and dentures (e.g. receding gums, ill-fitting dentures, peridontal disease, missing teeth).

2) **Respiratory:**
   — reduce immobility to a minimum: change position Q1-2H; encourage coughing and deep breathing to toleration;
   — maintain an environment conducive to adequate $O_2$ intake; reduce variables that decrease $O_2$ level; i.e. cigarette smoke, inadequate ventilation system;
   — observe and report symptoms of inadequate $O_2$ supply: blue nail beds, increased respirations, increased pulse rate, gasping; report early signs of URI.

3) **Gastrointestinal:**
   — ascertain which foods are tolerated by patient's digestive system; eliminate, or reduce to a minimum those which are poorly tolerated;
   — expect the time for eating and digestion to be increased; do not rush the patient—feed slowly; get orders for antacids PRN;
   — provide for dentures that are adequate or make sure food is in form that can be taken without dentures;
   — increase amount of flavoring and seasoning, if diagnosis and conditioning permit;
   — unless contraindicated, occasionally give candy to satisfy craving for sweets which is common in the aged;
   — observe for signs of constipation (no BM's for several days); report any problems to Dr.; give medications as prescribed;
   — ensure an adequate food and fluid intake.

**4) Musculoskeletal:**
— decrease in mineral metabolism (osteoporosis) causing changes in bone structure (often causes reduction in height, stooped posture, limits to mobility, brittle and easily broken bones);
— atrophy of skeletal muscles with a generalized decrease in strength, endurance and agility; muscles become flabby;
— changes in elastin & collagen fibers cause joint changes and immobility;
— patient fatigues easily;
— increase in curvature of spine.

**5) Genito-urinary:**
— 50% decrease in blood flow through kidneys, thus elimination of drugs through kidneys is impaired;
— diminished filtration rate and tubular function;
— increase in urinary incontinence;
— increase in frequency of urination;
— gradual atrophy of vaginal tissues; with a decrease in vaginal lubrication, size of uterus and cervix;
— enlargement of prostate.

**4) Musculoskeletal:**
— provide support for those persons who are unsteady (i.e. canes, walker, arm of nurse); allow patient to set pace for walking and other movements; s/he generally knows his abilities better than we do;
— do not expect patient to move as fast or accomplish tasks quickly, provide enough time;
— have firm-soled shoes or slippers for walking;
— encourage mild exercise; refer to NCPG #2:32, "Exercises for Patients Over 65";
— get pt. up & about at least Q2-3H to decrease stiffness and joint immobility;
— refer to NCPG #1:47, "ROM Exercises";
— be safety-conscious: prevent falls, remove obstacles, keep floors clean and dry, provide adequate lighting;
— keep bedrails in use and in good working order.

**5) Genito-urinary:**
— observe closely for signs & symptoms of overdose of drugs administered daily or frequently to patient; give meds. with sufficient fluids;
— provide periodic trips to BR or offer bedpan/urinal; use bedside commode or have male patients stand to void;
— if patient has difficulty with incontinence, provide protection for skin (Vaseline or Desitin), clothes, bedding; keep dry;
— refer to NCPG #2:03, "Bladder Retraining";
— if administering drugs through vaginal orifice, make sure a lubricant is utilized to ensure insertion and comfort.

6) **Endocrine:**
  — marked decrease in ability to fight disease;
  — increase in auto-immune properties;
  — increased susceptibility to disease, especially chronic disease;
  — decrease in glucose tolerance;
  — reduced production of gonadal hormones;
  — decrease production TSH—thyroid stimulating hormone & thyroid hormone.

7) **Nervous System:**
  — decreased blood supply & sclerotic changes in the brain cause cerebral deficits; signs include: confusion, loss of memory for recent events, lack of concentration, apathy, senility; (pseudo-senility can occur and is the symptomatic reflection of a self or other-imposed withdrawal from reality and/or isolation, not impaired circulation);
  — slowed reaction time;
  — decrease in visual acuity & accommodation to light;
  — loss of hearing of higher pitches;
  — decrease in number of taste buds;
  — slowed reflexes;

6) **Endocrine:**
  — observe & report promptly signs & symptoms of infection;
  — observe for diminished activity, fatigue;
  — protect patient from complications & infections; use good handwashing technique with each patient & when going from patient to patient; do not expose patient to others with infection or other communicable diseases, especially colds;
  — when caring for patient with infection, take vital signs for longer number of days since resistance to Rx increases with age;
  — do not expose patients to infections, colds you are carrying; stay home;
  — carefully remove bedding, clothing, etc. that may transfer germs from one area to another;
  — monitor intake of refined sugars.

7) **Nervous system:**
  — expect patient to ask you to repeat explanations, directions, questions; talk clearly, slowly and in plain language, repeating PRN; do not get angry at patient's inability to hear, or to discriminate words;
  — do not expect patient to accomplish tasks immediately or react quickly; provide more time for task accomplishment & for responding to spoken words; praise all efforts;
  — provide periodic opportunities for patient to express opinions, make choices/decisions re: occupational/recreational activities, care or needs;
  — sit down facing the patient when interacting with him in

order to prevent him from feeling rushed or pushed; talk clearly & slowly;

— do not assume that all problems are a result of physiology; observe behavioral responses to stimuli (see NCPG #2:26, "Common Behaviors"); assess environmental impact on patient; see NCPG #2:27, "Transition to Communal Living";

— provide for brighter lighting and color contrasts to increase discrimination & minimize glare; provide night lights;

— assess pain/discomfort in terms of individual tolerance levels, known or unknown ailments/diseases; refer to NCPG #1:30, "Pain."

8) **Skin:**
— dryness;
— loss of turgor, elasticity, hair;
— capillary fragility, bruises easily;
— diminished sense of touch & sensation;
— general thinning of epidermis;
— dermis loses strength & elasticity;
— loss of subcutaneous fat;
— change of hair color.

8) **Skin:**
— may need to have more blankets, higher thermostat level for heat;
— fewer baths (may not need a complete bath QD); use bath oils, emollient lotions PRN; avoid drying lotions, e.g. alcohol;
— use soft, unstarched bedsheets;
— avoid prolonged pressure over bony prominences; massage gently to increase circulation, prevent skin breakdown; change position at least Q2H;
— observe & report rashes, redness, cuts, lesions, drainage, itching & other abnormal skin conditions.

9) **Reproductive:**
— some modification of sexual capacity;
— loss of function due to lack of use.

9) **Reproductive:**
— desire for closeness and/or sexual activity should be encouraged and permitted.

**Recommended References**

"Common Skin Changes in the Elderly," by Diane Uhler. *American Journal of Nursing*, December 1976:1981–1982.

"Diabetes: Recommended Care of the Feet." NCP Guide #1:39, 2nd Ed., Nurseco, 1980.

"Drugs and the Elderly," by B. Gotz and V. Gotz. *American Journal of Nursing*, August 1978:1347–1351.

"Hazards of Immobility." NCP Guide #2:45, 2nd Ed., Nurseco, 1980.

"Physical Assessment, Parts A, B, C, D." NCP Guides #4:47, 48, 49, 50, Nurseco, 1978.

"Range of Motion Exercises." NCP Guide #1:47, 2nd Ed., Nurseco, 1980.

"Sex and the Elderly," by Winona Griggs. *American Journal of Nursing*, August 1978:1352–1354.

"Standards for Geriatric Nursing Practice," by ANA Division on Geriatric Nursing. *American Journal of Nursing*, September 1970:1894–1897.

"Supporting the Hospitalized, Elderly Person," by Ann Lore. *American Journal of Nursing*, March 1979:496–499.

"Symposium on Putting Geriatric Nursing Standards into Practice." *Nursing Clinics of North America*. Philadelphia, W.B. Saunders Company, June 1972:201–309.

"The Aged Patient: Common Behaviors." NCP Guide #2:26, 2nd Ed., Nurseco, 1980.

The Aged Patient: Exercises for Patients Over 65." NCP Guide #2:32, 2nd Ed., Nurseco, 1980.

"The Aged Patient: Transition to Communal Living." NCP Guide #2:27, 2nd Ed., Nurseco, 1980.

"The Cognitively Impaired Older Adult, by Miriam Hirschfield. *American Journal of Nursing*, December 1976:1981–1982.

"The Patient Experiencing Pain." NCP Guide #1:30, 2nd Ed., Nurseco, 1980.

"The Patient for Bladder Retraining." NCP Guide #2:03, 2nd Ed., Nurseco, 1980.

# Cast Care: General Principles

**LONG TERM GOAL:**   The patient will be clean, reasonably comfortable and safe from circulatory and nerve impairment within a cast whose purpose is maintained.

## General Considerations:
— Casts are applied to immobilize a body part in a specific position in order to: (a) correct or prevent a deformity, (b) provide rest and healing of a fracture, a soft tissue injury or bone infection, or (c) permit earlier weight-bearing of an injured body part.
— Nurses of orthopedic patients need to be expert in applying knowledge of body mechanics, functional body alignment, prevention of circulatory and nerve impairment, preservation of skin integrity and psychosocial adjustment of the confined patient. See NCPG #2:09, "The Patient with a Cast."

## Specific Considerations, Potential Patient Outcomes, and Nursing Actions:

1) Care of Wet Cast

The cast will be protected and supported in its original shape while it is drying and setting; optimal air will be circulated for evaporation of moisture without chilling or overheating patient:
— prepare orthopedic postop bed (see procedure manual) complete with bed board, firm mattress, overhead trapeze, footboard, bed cradle, sandbags, & extra pillows (towel-protected, cloth-covered—not rubber or plastic);
— use a cast dryer, hair dryer, fan or low wattage heat cradle according to surgeon's preference & unit policy;
— lift pt. (not roll or drop) in straight body alignment onto bed carefully & gently, while supporting cast with *palms* of hands; do not allow cast to sag unsupported at any point or to be impressed with fingerprints;
— support cast on soft pillows to prevent flattening; support remainder of pt. to prevent excessive weight on damp cast; keep heel (leg cast) elevated off mattress or pillow to prevent flat spot which could cause pressure;
— leave cast uncovered & provide good circulation of air; avoid drafts & prevent chills for pt.;
— turn pt. Q2H so all sides of cast will dry, supporting carefully both cast & pt.; have sufficient help to avoid injury to cast, pt. & lifting staff; instruct pt. & helpers in correct procedure for turning to the unaffected or unoperated side; replace damp pillows & sheets; plan on cast taking 24-48 hrs. to dry thoroughly (hip spica & body casts take longer);

2) Care of Dry Cast

The cast will be clean, dry, odor free and protected from damage:
— continue to support cast & pt. to maintain alignment, yet free of pressure on either cast or pt.;
— when cast is *thoroughly* dry, pull stockinette lining taut & fold back over edge of cast, trimming as needed & taping securely in place; if stockinette doesn't provide a smooth enough edge, pad slightly into sheet wadding or foam sponge;

then "petal" the cast edge with adhesive tape or moleskin sections (cut circle or diamond shaped); wet plaster of paris strips can be used to hold tape in place; rub to a smooth surface;

— *protect* the *entire cast* with a thin coat of polyurethane, "varnish" or shellac, brushed on (no spray cans, please); assure yourself & pt. of adequate ventilation during this process;

— *protect inside of cast* around buttocks & perineum from urine & fecal contamination; plastic wrap, sponge rubber, folded washcloths have been used with varying success; when placing pt. on bedpan, keep his shoulders higher than buttocks & wrap the edge of the cast with a dry towel to absorb quickly accidental spills;

— *clean stains* from outer cast with a sponge or cloth slightly dampened in a solution of Phisohex, benzalkonium chloride or other suitable deodorizing & antiseptic solution (non-alcohol to protect varnish seal); a small amt. of scouring cleanser may be used if necessary; then quickly rub, fan or blow dry dampened area of cast;

— *clean inside edges of cast* by removing wet or soiled sheet wadding or stockinette; replace with a similar, soft, absorbent material; replace waterproof wrapping PRN; to prevent mold & musty odors, be sure cast is dry before covering it again;

— use new layers of plaster to "patch" or refurbish cast; it must be skillfully applied & rubbed smoothly into place or it may peel off later; dry new plaster addition quickly & thoroughly.

**3) Removal of Cast**

The cast will be removed safely without injury or discomfort to patient; the cast will be removed carefully and undamaged if it needs to be reused as a splint or temporary "shell":

— explain & reassure pt. that s/he'll feel only vibration of saw & some heat;

— have all necessary equipment (cast cutter, "spreaders," etc.) on hand for surgeon or asst. who will remove cast;

— the cast may be softened with towels soaked in a mild vinegar & water solution for half an hour prior to cutting, if the cast is to be discarded;

— if cast is to be bi-valved & reused, be prepared to replace padded lining and stockinette; massage pt.'s skin with emollient lotion & allow to dry completely before carefully replacing the plaster "halves" or "splints"; wrap entire cast with elastic bandage to hold cast in correct position.

**Recommended References**

"Casts, Your Patients & You—Part I—A Review of Basic Procedures: Cast Application, Cast Management, Cast Wearing & Removal," by Jane Farrell. *Nursing '78*, October 1978:65–69.
"The Patient with a Cast." NCP Guide #2:09, 2nd Ed., Nurseco, 1980.

# Crisis Intervention: Adaptation to General Nursing

**GOAL:** The patient will regain at least his pre-crisis level of functioning; *or* (if the crisis has not yet occurred) the patient will respond adaptively to the loss and maintain emotional equilibrium.

**General Considerations:**
— **Dynamics of a crisis:**
  - A stress or life change event can cause a real or anticipated *loss* or losses in an individual (Review NCPG #1:31, "Responses to Loss . . .").
  - This loss creates a *hazard* (or hazardous situation) for the patient which *can* develop into a crisis.
  - A *precipitating event* pushes the patient from a hazard into a crisis, and may be major or minor; often it is the "last straw."
  - A *crisis* is the emotional response to a hazard, and occurs when the patient is unable to resolve the loss (or losses) because his usual coping mechanisms aren't working or are unavailable, and the patient is said to be in a state of disequilibrium or instability.
— Nurses in general care units most often see patients in a hazardous situation rather than in a state of crisis.
— **Types** of hazards:
  1) *Situational:* Relates to areas of daily living, e.g. physical illness; change in usual role/job; divorce/separation/retirement.
  2) *Maturational:* relates to a person's developmental tasks, e.g. puberty; adolescence; adulthood; onset of menopause; old age.

**Assessment:**
— The **Aguilera model** for assessment of a hazard or a crisis is based on 3 balancing factors:
  1) *Realistic perception of what is/has happened:* What does it mean to the patient? Is the perception realistic or not?
  2) *Adequate situational supports:* Does the patient have family, friends, someone s/he can trust? Someone with whom s/he can talk?
  3) *Adequate coping mechanisms:* What does the patient usually do to cope with stress (talk to someone? go to a movie? work? drugs? alcohol?). Almost anything, in moderation, is adaptive; in excess, it is probably maladaptive.
— If 2 of these 3 balancing factors are present, the patient is probably in a hazardous situation (rather than a true crisis), and a crisis *very likely will not occur.*

**Intervention:**
— Intervention is based on assessment of the balancing factors and is aimed at restoring and strengthening them by:
  — correcting unrealistic perceptions;

— providing adequate situational supports; and

— helping the patient find alternate coping mechanisms.

— **Types of intervention:**

1) *General support:* consists of listening to the patient, allowing him to talk at length and in detail about what is bothering him; *not* challenging any of his statements; and staying with him. This kind of support is usually begun on initial contact, during assessment and helps you determine the patient's perception of what is happening to him (balancing factor #1). When the patient's behavior indicates that he is beginning to adapt or cope (begins to focus on reality; ask questions), support and reinforce reality, answer questions honestly, share with patient how you see it, and ask him to clarify or validate your perceptions.

2) *Environmental manipulation:* consists of changing factors in the environment to help lower the acute stress/anxiety; and providing adequate situational supports (balancing factor #2): e.g. flexing visiting hours; moving patient to another room; use of TV, telephone; a warm bath, back rub. Ask the patient what he thinks would help him right now; if at all possible, provide it.

3) *Generic approach:* based on knowledge of responses to a loss (the Grief and Mourning Process), intervention is geared toward adaptive resolution of the hazard/crisis. This approach can help the patient find new coping mechanisms or ways of restoring old ones that have been temporarily unavailable.

4) *Individual approach:* based on knowledge and application of intrapsychic and interpersonal processes, intervention is planned around the unique needs of the patient in a specific crisis. This approach is used appropriately by mental health workers only.

**Implications for the nurse:**

Knowledge of crisis intervention will help reduce a nurse's feelings of helplessness when confronted with a patient in crisis; she will be able to help the patient and/or family *maintain* emotional equilibrium (in a hazardous situation) or *regain it* (in a crisis state). How?

— She will know that by providing general and environmental support, she will be reducing the patient's level of anxiety and stress so that he can begin to cope with what is happening to him.

— Assessment of the three balancing factors will tell her where the deficits/gaps are and thus which ones to restore and/or strengthen.

— She will know that the first two types of intervention can be provided by *any* care giver, and that they will be provided frequently, for varying lengths of time, throughout the day or night.

— She will know that a higher level of intervention can be provided by the generic approach for which knowledge of the Grief and Mourning Process is essential.

**Evaluation:**
— Where a nurse has provided this type of nursing care, is there a way she can *evaluate* and *validate* the interventions prescribed? Yes. How?
— Ask the patient. Ask him, "What kinds of things made you feel better?" "Was there anything else that might have helped?" You may find that some of the most helpful things were simply being with the patient; allowing him to cry, etc.
— For application of this information, see NCPG #2:31, "The Patient Needing Crisis Intervention."

**Recommended References**

*Crisis Intervention* by Donna Aguilera and Janice Messick, 2nd Ed. St. Louis: The C.V. Mosby Co.: 1974.

"The Patient Needing Crisis Intervention." NCP Guide #2:31, 2nd Ed., Nurseco, 1980.

"Responses to Loss: the Grief and Mourning Process." NCP Guide #1:31, 2nd Ed., Nurseco, 1980.

# Drugs: Asthma

**GOAL:**  The patient will use prescribed drugs effectively to prevent, relieve, and control asthmatic attacks.

**General Considerations:**
— Drugs play a major role in symptomatic treatment of acute asthmatic attacks. Some are also given to liquefy secretions and keep the tracheo-bronchial tree patent.
— **Nursing responsibilities** include:
  • knowing the actions, usual dosages, untoward side effects, and nursing implications for each prescribed drug;
  • administering each drug as ordered, including questioning of and verifying with Dr. any dose that a nurse considers questionable as to safety, etc.;
  • charting patient responses to the drugs and notifying Dr. of any untoward side effects; and
  • teaching actions, dosages, and side effects of drugs to the patient and family as preparation for discharge.

| Drug Type & Examples | Actions | Side Effects & Nursing Implications |
|---|---|---|
| **Bronchodilator** | | |
| *Adrenalin* | Relieves spasm rapidly; effect of short duration | Side effects are common and include palpitation, tachycardia, tremors, pallor, anxiety; check vital signs Q15-30 mins.; stay with patient. |
| *Aminophylline* | Slow, prolonged effect | Given slowly to avoid sudden drop in BP; dizziness, faintness, palpitation, headache, irritability; as above; never given with epinephrine, or ephedrine unless dosage reduced, otherwise it potentiates toxic effect. |
| *Ephedrine* | Takes 20 mins. to be effective; lasts longer than epinephrine; relieves nocturnal paroxymsm and wheezing related to exercise | Nervousness, trembling, insomnia, tachycardia; do not give with Aminophylline (see above). |
| *Isuprel* | Aerosol use only | Palpitations, anginal pain, nervousness, tremor, headache, nausea |

**Detergent**

| | | |
|---|---|---|
| *Alevaire* | Helps keep airways clear | None |

**Anti-inflammatory Agent**

| | | |
|---|---|---|
| *Corticosteroids (Prednisone)* | Given on long-term basis, helps prevent recurring attacks | GI bleeding; hemorrhage, moonface, Na. retention, hirsutism, N&V, diarrhea; observe for & report signs of bleeding, edema; keep accurate I&O. |

**Expectorant**

| | | |
|---|---|---|
| *Ammonium Chloride* | Helps thin thick secretions; mild diuretic | If taken in large amounts over long period of time, possible GI upset; do not give with milk; push fluids. |
| *Potassium Iodide (saturated solution)* | As above | May have an effect on existing thyroid problems or glaucoma. |
| **Sedatives & Tranquilizers** | Many, many available and used (see NCPG #3:45, 47); help control anxiety during an attack | Drug dependency; respiratory failure; avoid alcohol when taking. |

**Recommended References**
"Drugs: Tranquilizers." NCP Guide #3:47, Nurseco, 1977.
"Drugs, Hypnotics and Sedatives." NCP Guide #3:45, Nurseco, 1977.
"Over-the-Counter Bronchodilators," by Joan E. Webber-Jones and Melanie K. Bryant. *Nursing '80*, January 1980:34–39.
*Physicians' Desk Reference*. Oradell, N.J.: Medical Economics, current issue.
"What to Watch for with Minor Tranquilizers," by Sara White and Karin Williamson. *RN*, November 1979:57–59.

# Drugs: Cardiac

**GOALS:**  The patient will have a reduction of and control over symptoms of cardiac dysfunction; will have strengthened and improved cardiac output and will maintain electrolyte balance.

## General Considerations:
— Although several drugs are commonly used by many physicians and hospitals, many others are available; drug choice, dosage, route of administration are highly variable, and depend on the Dr., condition and status of the patient, as well as protocol of the unit (if an ICU or CCU); check orders carefully.
— Familiarize yourself with the pharmaceutical literature accompanying the drugs; know the side effects, toxic manifestations, actions and usual dosages of each one.
— **Nursing responsibilities** in drug therapy are to medicate the patient as ordered (but always stopping short of what s/he believes to be unsafe dosages), observe and chart patient response to drugs, report side effects to Dr., explain purpose, action, side effects of drug to patient, and enlist patient's cooperation in this form of treatment.

## Drug Type & Action

| Cardiac Depressants<br>Nursing Implications | Side Effects/Toxic Reactions | Nursing Implications |
| --- | --- | --- |
| *Xylocaine (Lidocaine)*<br>Rapid acting (45-90 sec.); depresses ventricular excitability; good for PVCs | Mild euphoria; muscle twitching; blurred vision; sensation of heat, cold, numbness; discomfort with speaking, swallowing, convulsions, hypotension | Check monitor for PVCs; ensure against over-infusion of I/V drip; check concentration given. |
| *Pronestyle (Procaine amide)*<br>Used in treatment of PVCs and ventricular tachycardia; decrease cardiac irritability | Hypotension; hypersensitivity to chills & fever; weakness, skin rash, N&V; diarrhea | Monitor BP; provide extra blankets PRN; if patient nauseated, have him take some deep breaths and exhale slowly; offer small sips of carbonated fluids, weak tea; observe for rash. |

*Quinidine:* used for ectopic rhythms, atrial tachycardia, flutter & fibrillation, ventricular tachycardia, premature systoles; slows conduction time in atrium

Decreased BP; respiratory distress; convulsions; A-V & cardiac asystole; ventricular fibrillation; diarrhea, N&V, dizziness, headache, ringing in ears

Monitor vital signs Q2-4H; contraindicated in complete heart block.

*Digoxin (Lanoxin)*
Rapid acting; initial effect IV in 5-10 mins.; strengthens cardiac contractions, slows the rate, thus increasing cardiac output

N&V, anorexia, headache, visual disturbances, cardiac dysrhythmias, headache, fatigue, malaise, drowsiness; pulse below 60, irregular & intermittent rate; A-V block

Take pulse before giving med.; withhold if pulse below 60; be especially alert to signs of digitalis toxicity in elderly patients as they tolerate the drug poorly; a slight drop in serum potassium level (below 4.4 mEq./L) can cause signs of digitalis toxicity; check lab. reports of serum potassium; provide foods high in K (see NCPG #2:48, "Potassium Imbalance").

*Cedilanid-D*
A rapid-acting digitalis preparation

Same as Digoxin

Same as Digoxin

*G-Strophantin (Quabain)*
Same effect as Digoxin; usually given IV for rapid digitalization; used for patients who need digitalis but do not respond to that drug

Same as Digoxin

Same as Digoxin

*Propranolol HCL (Inderal)*
Used to control ventricular response to atrial fibrillation, flutter, or tachycardia; to treat angina

Not to be given to patients with A-V block or CHF

Monitor response; make sure patient has no history of asthma or COPD.

**Bretylium Tosylate (Bretylol)**
Treat ventricular tachycardia and ventricular fibrillation which do not respond to Lidocaine, Quinidine or Procainamide

Potentiates digitalis-induced dysrhythmias; may increase hypotensive effects of Quinidine and Propanolol; N&V

Monitor P, BP after administration; assure patient that side effects relate to rapid administration of drug.

**Norpace**
Treat PVCs and prevent ventricular tachycardia

Urinary retention and hesitancy; dryness of mucous membranes; nausea, gas pains, constipation; fatigue, headache, SOB, hypotension

Monitor bodily response to drug; take vital signs frequently; inform patient that side effects may occur and to discuss body changes with you.

**Edrophonium (Tensilon)**
Used to treat atrial tachycardia

Bradycardia, cardiac standstill; hypotension, weakness, convulsions; increased bronchial secretions; respiratory paralysis

Increase frequency of monitoring patient's vital signs, especially P, R, BP; explain to patient that s/he should call a nurse if experiencing any changes in how s/he feels.

## Cardiac Stimulants
**Atropine**
Causes an increase in heart rate; reduces degree of A-V block

Dryness of mouth; blurred vision; restlessness; confusion; hallucinations; increased BP; difficulty in voiding; PVCs; decreased bronchial secretions; contraindicated in glaucoma and tachycardia

Check pulse; withhold med. if patient has tachycardia; safety precautions PRN (side rails, sitter); check voiding.

**Epinephrine (Adrenalin)**
Improves myocardial contractions and rhythmicity; often injected directly into heart in cardiac arrest; increases pulse & BP; reduces degree of heart block

Increased nervousness, muscular tremor, anxiety, ventricular fibrillation; reduced urinary output; angina, headache

Assure patient that these uncomfortable feelings are temporary; check P & BP at least Q15 mins.

*Isuprel*
A bronchodilator and smooth muscle relaxant; produces an increase in cardiac output

**Electrolyte Solutions/Alkalizers**
*Sodium Bicarbonate*
Reverses metabolic acidosis; and respiratory acidosis (from $CO_2$ retention)

*Potassium Chloride*
Helps suppress cardiac irritability & dysrhythmias, especially in digitalis toxicity; corrects potassium deficit

**Anticoagulants**
*Heparin*
Parenteral drug for immediate anticoagulant action; used for prophylaxis and treatment of thrombi/ emboli.

Flushing of face, sweating, mild tremor or sensation of pounding in chest; hypotension; dysrhythmias; PVCs, sinus tachycardia, ventricular tachycardia or fibrillation.

Depressed respirations; muscle hypertoxicity; hyperactive reflexes, tetany; possible convulsions; alkalosis

Hyperkalemia; EKG changes, cardiac arrest; renal insufficiency; GI disturbances; vein irritation, bradycardia; depression of pacemaker cells

Bleeding at injection site; generally non-toxic effects are immediate & quickly dissipated, and are promptly reversible, if needed, with protamine sulphate.

Not to be given with Adrenalin, although the two drugs may be given alternately; assure patient that side effects are temporary.

Monitor respirations; prevent over-infusion of IV; incompatible with most other drugs; don't add meds. to IV solution.

Concentrated solutions must be diluted before administering to prevent hyperkalemia and development of lesions in the intestines; be alert to signs of hyperkalemia (malaise, weakness, mental confusion, slowed pulse); keep an accurate I&O; monitor apical pulse.

Observe and chart signs of *external bleeding* (gums, urine, rectum); have injectable vitamin K & protamine sulphate available as antidotes; observe & chart signs of *internal bleeding* (faintness, weakness, inc. pulse, dec. BP, black & blue marks); check orders for daily prothrombin time order (drug dosage is regulated according to the results); clotting time determinations are usually done by lab.

*Warfarin, Sodium (Doumadin)*
Used for long term anticoagulant therapy to prevent sudden, acute arterial occlusion.

Hemorrhage, due to hypothrombinemia; actions *potentiated* by Quinidine, thyroid drugs, salicylates, Edecrin, Phenylbutazone, Chloramphenical; *inhibited* by adrenocortical steroids, barbiturates, Meprobamate

before each IV infusion; injections are usually given SC or intrafat, as IM ones cause pain, hematoma, delay onset of action & create a shorter duration of effect. If patient discharged on anticoagulant therapy, ensure that s/he knows to report any bleeding, weakness or dizziness to Dr., and has a written dosage schedule.

Same as for Heparin.

*Dicumeral*
Used in acute MI to prevent extension of clot and formation of mural thrombi; does not resolve thrombi and emboli already formed.

Hematuria; bleeding from mucous membranes, wound or ulcerative lesions, bruises; contraindicated for patients with active TB, hypertension, liver or kidney disease, history of ulcers; same potentiating and inhibiting effects as Warfarin, Sodium

Same as Heparin; promptly report vomiting, diarrhea or fever because these can affect absorption and metabolism of drug.

## Diuretics
*Furosemide (Lasix)*
A potent, short-acting diuretic (5 mins. via IV; first hour orally); effects are short-lived (2 hrs. for IV; 6-8 hrs. orally); blocks reabsorption of sodium

Excessive amounts can lead to water and electrolyte depletion; N&V, diarrhea, skin rash, pruritis, blurred vision

Give drug in am; weigh daily, keep accurate I&O; check serum K level & observe for signs of hypokalemia (general malaise, apathy, weakness, muscle cramps, dizziness on rising, mental confusion); provide foods high in potassium (see NCPG #2:48); be alert to postural hypotension.

| Thiazides (Diuril, Hydrodiuril) | | |
|---|---|---|
| Most widely-used diuretics; used for CHF, retention of sodium due to steroid therapy; inhibit reabsorption of sodium, water & chloride in kidney tubules | Same as Furosemide | Same as Furosemide |

**Recommended References**

"Antiarrhythmic Drug Therapy," by Janet Stanford, Joel Felner and Daniel Arensberg. *American Journal of Nursing*, July 1980:1288–1295.

"Digitalis" by Elizabeth H. Winslow. *American Journal of Nursing*, June 1974:1062–1065.

"How Patient Education Can Reduce the Risks of Anticoagulation," by Karen Moore and Barbara J. Maschak. *Nursing '77*, September 1977:24–29.

"Keeping Anticoagulants Under Control," by John Hand. *RN*, April 1979:25–29.

*Memory Bank for Critical Care*, by Gary Ervin. Pacific Palisades, CA: Nurseco, 1979.

"The Effect of Antianginal Drugs on Myocardial Oxygen Consumption," by Ellen Fuller. *American Journal of Nursing*, February 1980:250–254.

# Drugs: Parkinson's Disease

**LONG TERM GOALS:** The patient's disease symptoms will be reduced and controlled; the patient will recognize and understand undesirable but common side effects; serious complications and untoward reactions will be prevented; appropriate dosage levels will be determined with the collaboration of patient, family, nurse and physician.

**General Considerations:**
— Drug dosage varies considerably according to individual symptoms and severity of disease, personal tolerance levels, general health status, and the synergistic activity when two or more drugs are used in combination.
— **Nursing responsibility** rests with teaching patient as needed to enlist his help in identifying side effects and expected drug effectiveness; careful observation and recording of all signs and symptoms of desirable as well as undesirable drug actions; and provision of nursing measures designed to enhance the drug's effectiveness while minimizing its untoward effects.

| Drug Type & Action | Examples | Side Effects | Nursing Implications |
| --- | --- | --- | --- |
| **Levodopa**<br>— converted into dopamine both inside & outside brain;<br>— relieves P.D. symptoms in most patients | *L-Dopa*<br>*Dopar*<br>*Larodopa*<br>*Benodopa* | anorexia, N/V,<br>dry mouth, burning sensation of tongue,<br>constipation,<br>diarrhea,<br>GI bleeding,<br>dizziness, changes in alertness (increase or decrease),<br>occasional increase in sexual arousal,<br>depression<br><br>urine may turn red | — take with meals.<br>— give pt. hard candy, lozenges or gum.<br>— urge fruits & fruit juices for constipation.<br>— observe for tarry stools.<br>— avoid driving or operating machinery.<br>— explain to pt./family.<br>— report severe depression or suicidal tendencies.<br>— tell pt./family this is harmless. |

| | |
|---|---|
| abnormal, involuntary movements (dyskinesia) such as pouting, grimacing, tongue movements, twisting of neck, arms or legs | — help pt./family to accept this expected effect. |
| rapid blinking of eyes | — may be early sign of overdose. |
| orthostatic hypotension | — have pt. wear elastic stockings, change positions slowly, lie down when feeling faint. |
| cardiac dysrhythmias L-dopa absorbed in fat deposits | — have overweight pts. lose weight to facilitate effective dosage management & to reduce cardiovascular problems. |
| effects antagonized by alcohol | — limit intake of alcohol to one drink per day. |
| effects diminished by pyridoxine and by high protein intake | — limit intake of $B_6$ to 5 mg. per day; avoid multivitamin dosages.<br>— limit intake of meat, milk, eggs, fish, cheese & poultry & spread mod. amts. of protein throughout meals of day. |

| | | | |
|---|---|---|---|
| **Levidopa and Carbidopa**<br>— blocks dopamine production<br>outside brain | *Sinamet* | curtails GI & cardiac side effects, reduces dizziness & fainting effects of L-Dopa | |
| | | not necessary to limit pyridoxine intake | |
| | | dyskinesias may appear at lower dosage levels | |
| | | other side effects similar to dopamine | — refer to nursing implications above. |
| **Antiviral Agent**<br>**Amantadine**<br>— releases dopamine at storage sites | *Symmetrel* | swelling of feet | — have pt. elevate feet when sitting. |
| | | possible blood clot release, bone fracture | — safety precautions.<br>— observe for thrombophlebitis, pulmonary embolus. |
| | | depressions, psychotic reactions | — observe & record unusual behavior. |
| | | orthostatic hypotension | — same as aforementioned.<br>— watch for loss of effect after 3-6 mos. admin. |
| **Anticholinergics**<br>— parasympathetic inhibitors, blocking effect of acetylcholine, decrease salivation, improve muscle control | *Artane*<br>*Kemadrin*<br>*Pagitane*<br>*Akineton*<br>*Pipadol* | dry mouth<br>blurred vision<br>constipation<br>difficulty voiding | — give pt. candy or gum.<br>— safety precautions.<br>— check elimination & take corrective measures.<br>— increase fluids.<br>— watch for loss of effectiveness after 3-6 mos. admin. |

| **Antihistamines**<br>— used alone as initial therapy<br>  for milder symptoms<br>— relieves rigidity, sedates, anti-<br>  depressant | *Benadryl*<br>*Disipal*<br>*Histol*<br>*Phenoxene* | drowsiness,<br>dizziness<br>nausea<br>dry mouth | — same as above mentioned. |
| **Combination of above two types**<br>**in actions** | *Cogentin*<br>*Parsidol*<br>*Panparnit*<br>*Toryn* | same as above | — same as above. |

**Recommended References**

"Do's and Don'ts for the Patient on Levodopa Therapy," by Rebecca Langan and George Cotzias. *American Journal of Nursing*, June 1976:917,918.

"The Whats and Whys of Drug Therapy in Parkinsonism," by Frances Fischbach. *American Journal of Nursing*, January 1978:67.

# Catheters: Indwelling Urethral

**GOAL:** A properly functioning urinary drainage system will be established and maintained; cystitis and more serious infection complications will be prevented from developing.

**General Considerations:**
— Indwelling catheters should be used only when absolutely necessary:
  (a) for incontinence when all other measures have failed;
  (b) for paralytic bladders and the use of a tidal drainage program;
  (c) for intermittent drainage of obstructed or overdistended bladders;
  (d) for protection of an operative area from urine or pressure of bladder distention; and
  (e) to monitor urine output during treatment of shock, burns or critical care patients.
— Daily urine output of normal adult is 1200-1500 ml.; specific gravity range: 1.010-1.025; pH: 4.8-8.5 (avg. 6, slightly acid).
— While the bladder is normally resistant to inflammation and infection, when a catheter is left in for more than a few hours, the chances of bacteriuria are greatly increased. Most infections are caused by Escherichia coli, Klebsiella, Aerobacter, Pseudomonas, and Proteus organisms normally found on the skin or in the hospital environment. According to the Center for Disease Control, about 40% of all hospital-acquired infections occur in the urinary tract; about ¾ of these are attributed to indwelling catheters. Rigid aseptic technique with the catheter drainage unit is therefore essential.
— Individual attitudes and behaviors regarding elimination vary. These should be recognized and accepted in order to maintain a therapeutic nurse-patient relationship.

**Specific Considerations, Potential Patient Outcomes, and Nursing Actions:**
1) Infection Control
The formation of calculi will be retarded; bacterial growth and nosocomial infection will be prevented; normal urine composition, specific gravity, and pH will be maintained:
  — wash hands thoroughly before handling pt. or equipment;
  — use only sealed, sterile units (catheter, drainage tube & collection container); employ strict aseptic technique; wear sterile gloves; cleanse perineum with iodophor solution; use antibacterial lubricant (eg. Lubrasporin) on catheter tip and meatus before insertion;
  — change catheter & complete unit only when necessary for accumulated sediment or leakage (avg. 1 to 4 weeks); however, frequent intermittent catheterization with sterile technique has also been found to have a reduced rate of infections;

— place 100 ml. of 20-40% Formaldehyde in collection unit (by syringe . . . don't disconnect!);

— cleanse perineum at least twice daily with mild soap and water; rinse & dry thoroughly; apply neomycin-polymyxin B ointment around meatus;

— ensure a fluid intake to 2500-3000 ml. daily (unless contraindicated); know that a urinary flow of at least 25 ml./hour keeps bacteria flowing downward & retards sediment formation in tube;

— give cranberry or prune juice, 200-400 ml. daily, to promote a slightly acid urine, helping to prevent calcium phosphate stones; other acid ash foods include eggs, meat, poultry, cereal corn, prunes, plums; if pt. is on streptomycin, sulfonamide or inversine therapy, an alkaline urine is desirable; then give orange juice, citrus fruits, vegetables while reducing intake of acid ash foods previously listed;

— obtain urine specimens with sterile 25 g. needle and 5 ml. syringe; after cleansing rubber with antiseptic swab, insert with a slant into a flared or distal end of catheter; send to lab in sterile tube;

— *never disconnect catheter from drainage unit unless absolutely necessary;* transport or ambulate pt. with closed unit intact; when disconnection is unavoidable, use sterile catheter plug & discard after single usage; before emptying drainage bag, wipe spigot with alcohol sponge; do not let the spigot touch anything else;

— when irrigations are needed more than once daily; use a three-way catheter or connecting Y-tube to establish a closed, overhead irrigation system with antibacterial solution;

— instruct pt./family in catheter care, hand-washing & prevention of contamination.

2) Effective
   Functioning

Gravity flow drainage will be assured without backflow into bladder, blockage of flow or interruption of closed system; the privacy, reasonable comfort and acceptance by the patient will be ensured:

— tape (non-irritating type) catheter to inside of pt.'s thigh, placing drainage tube between or under legs, & securing it to bed linen at side of bed, allowing pt. freedom of movement;

— keep drainage tube descending directly to collection unit without any dependent loops causing urine to move uphill slowly before flowing into container;

— keep collection unit & tubing covered by sheets; ease of visibility to a passing nurse is not more important than preventing pt.'s embarrassment;

— check on urinary output & patency of drainage system Q2H; explain the system to pt. enlisting cooperation of pt. when able;

— note sediment build-up, mucous shreds, blood clots or stones which impede flow; irrigation may be necessary to clear blockage if "milking" tube doesn't work; use sterile equipment & sterile technique; slow, gentle infusion of room temperature solution reduces likelihood of bladder spasms & pt. discomfort;
— clamp tubing whenever collection unit is lifted to the height of the mattress, such as when turning pt. or moving by litter; preferably keep collection unit below bladder level at all times; hang bag at the correct level in a sling attached to the litter or back of wheelchair in transporting pt.; instruct pt./family in prevention of reflux.

3) Observations  Accurate, pertinent information will be recorded; impending complications will be recognized via early, warning signs:
— observe & record color, odor, amt. & appearance of urine each time collection unit is emptied;
— determine specific gravity & pH of urine collected one hour after collection has been previously emptied; note time of day;
— record accurately total intake & output Q8H;
— report pt. complaints of burning, irritation, low abdominal distention or pressure, chills, fever, flank pain, etc.

4) Catheter    Normal muscle tone and function of the bladder will be maintained as much as possible:
   Removal   — plan & implement periodic clamping of catheter for 2-3 hr. intervals for at least two days before removing catheter;
— tidal drainage may be used to facilitate returning bladder control or an "automatic" bladder;
— see NCPG #2:03, "The Patient for Bladder Retraining."

**Recommended References**
"Intermittent Self Catheterization," by Martha Hartman. *Nursing '78*, November 1978:72–75.
"The Patient for Bladder Retraining." NCP Guide #2:03, 2nd Ed., Nurseco, 1980.
"You Can Improve Your Catheterized Patient's Care," by Luanne Bellfy. *RN*, April 1977:33–35.

## Central Venous Pressure Line (CVP)

**Definition:**   CVP is a measurement of pressure in the superior vena cava, indicating the competency of the right heart.

**Purposes:**   A CVP line is often used in acute situations to:
- measure the relationship between blood volume and cardiac competency
- monitor and administer IV fluids and drugs
- provide a route for placement of an endocardial pacemaker electrode
- permit withdrawal of blood
- indicate status and response of patient to treatment

**Procedure:**   The CVP line can be connected to a transducer or oscilloscope, but is *usually* connected to a water manometer. Most of these are pre-packaged and disposable; thoroughly familiarize yourself with guides and instructions on package, or with other set-up in your facility.

Explain procedure to patient, giving as much information as s/he wants: purposes, what s/he can expect in terms of pain, discomfort, etc.

Prepare manometer by filling it with IV solution to the 10 cm. level (Keep IV tubing attached via stopcock, in closed position.)

Secure manometer to IV pole so that the zero mark is level with patient's mid-axillary line (level of right atrium) when patient is lying flat. Mark this level on patient's chest; this ensures a constant base line.

A catheter is passed (by a Dr.) into the tip of the SVC, usually via an arm or neck vein, and connected to the manometer via the stopcock (in a closed position) and taped securely to patient.

**To Take a Reading:**   Readings should be taken with patient in *same* position each time, preferably flat in bed unless his condition contraindicates:
- check to see that manometer is filled with solution to the 10 cm. level and that zero mark is level with patient's atrium (mark on patient's chest);
- turn stopcock to permit IV solution in manometer to flow into patient's vein;
- observe drop in fluid level in manometer; level will fall until it balances CVP in the SVC. This new level indicates the CVP in cm. of water.

Readings may be taken continuously or intermittently. If the latter, keep stopcock turned so that IV solution does not flow through manometer in-between readings.

The **normal CVP measurement is 3-10 cm. water.** *An abrupt rise in CVP* may indicate, among others, onset of a cardiac dysrhythmia, misplaced catheter, right ventricular failure, increased blood volume, pulmonary embolism, obstruction of the line. *A low CVP reading* may indicate hypovolemia, dehydration, disconnected CVP line.

**Is Your Reading Valid?**
To ensure a valid reading, check the following:
1) When you turn stopcock to permit manometer fluid to run into patient's vein, does level fall rapidly? (It should)
2) Does fluid level in manometer fluctuate with respirations, and rise sharply when patient coughs? (It should)
3) Can you aspirate blood from line? (Should be able to do this)
To ensure patency, CVP line should be flushed intermittently with a dilute solution of Heparin; consult physician for amount.

**Maintenance:**
Nursing responsibilities and goals include prevention of infection and malposition of catheter.

Refer to NCPG #2:46 (IV Therapy), section on "Specific Considerations . . ." for measures to prevent infection and preserve catheter site.

Malposition of the catheter may be caused by initial misplacement, migration, or advancement of tip when patient moves. Caution patient against sudden movements or applying pressure to line; ensure that line/catheter are taped securely to patient.

**Recommended References**
"CVP Monitoring," by Joy Murray and Janet Smallwood. *Nursing 77,* January 1977:42–47.
"Intravenous Therapy: General Principles." NCP Guide #2:46, 2nd Ed., Nurseco, 1980.

# General Postoperative Nursing Care, Part A:
## Support of Pulmonary Functions

**LONG TERM GOAL:** The patient will regain consciousness, reestablish normal physiological functioning and adapt psychologically to the trauma of surgery and its consequences; the postop surgical patient will recover successfully, free of preventable complications.

**General Considerations:**

— Patients having abdominal, thoracic or pelvic surgery under general anesthesia require competent nursing care postoperatively to restore normal functioning of all body systems free of preventable complications. For total care refer to specific considerations, nursing actions, and references in NCPG #2:42, "Support of Cardiovascular, Genitourinary, and Gastrointestinal Functions," and NCPG #2:43, "Support of Auxiliary Functions."

— Most patients go to a Recovery Room or Intensive Care Unit until they have regained consciousness, have stable vital signs and are in satisfactory condition to be returned to the surgical nursing units.

— For those patients who return to the surgical unit directly from OR, remember,

(1) the patient's hearing is the first sense to resume functioning; monitor your voice and speech to reduce patient's fright and distorted perceptions;

(2) all patients should be routinely checked and assessed the first 72 hours with this frequency; Q15min. × 4, Q30min. × 4, Q1H × 4, then Q4H and *more* often when encountering an unfavorable sign;

(3) determine the type of anesthetic agent used and its expected side effects on patient during the recovery phase; have suitable antagonist meds. on hand;

(4) determine the nature and outcome of surgery and consult surgeon or anesthesiologist for information about any unusual occurrence (shock, hemorrhage, cardiac arrest, dysrhythmias, trauma caused by equipment or positioning, etc.) which may affect the patient's condition or recovery period;

(5) review the patient's admission history and pre-operative nursing assessment record for factors that will affect the recovery process; eg, allergies, presence of a pacemaker, cough or URI, history of smoking, infections, rashes, special emotional concerns (fear of surgery, of death, of diagnosis), physical limitations, etc.; refer to NCPG #2:44, "General Preoperative Nursing Care"; *and*

(6) locate family/friends in attendance and keep them regularly informed about the patient's condition and progress. Give them a chance to ask questions, to express concerns, to see the patient, and to be reassured that all is being done for the patient that is needed.

**Specific Considerations, Potential Patient Outcomes, and Nursing Actions:**

1) Pulmonary Function

The patient will have normal respiratory function within three days postop; the patient will maintain adequate ventilation and a patent airway; accumulated bronchial secretions will be removed; the patient will have clear lungs and be free of preventable complications: hypoxia, atelectasis and pneumonia:

— assess patency of airway and adequacy of ventilation; take corrective actions judged needed;

— monitor & record TPR & BP, at least as often as ordered, noting quality & changes, assessing significance & reporting accordingly;

— retain pharyngeal or tracheal airway until coughing & swallowing reflexes have returned, the pt. can lift own head from bed & the pt. is adequately ventilating self as determined by your judgment, by spirometer measurements &/or by arterial blood gas determinations (norms: pH 7.35-7.45, $PaO_2$ 80-100 mm Hg, Pa $CO_2$ 35-45 mm Hg);

— suction pharynx & trachea PRN; use gloves & sterile catheter each time & give $O_2$ before & after 10 second suctioning sessions, allowing pt. to rest;

— observe closely for respiratory tract obstructions (edema, blood, mucus plugs, vomit, tongue); keep head to side to prevent regurgitation; note & report restlessness & rapid, thready pulse (early signs), snoring, gasping, apprehension, cyanosis, apnea, retraction;

— observe any abnormal respiratory pattern: "crowing," "wheezing," aberrant movements or altered behavior; report to MD STAT;

— watch for "splinting" & shallow breathing caused by incisional pain &/or too tight dressing; give medications as ordered PRN for pain & nausea, but observe closely for respiratory depression;

— position when possible in a side lying position, with head & neck slightly hyperextended; turn or change position at least Q1H first 8 postoperative hours, then at least Q2H for as long as the pt. remains bedfast & unable to turn self;

— observe pt. perform deep breathing exercises at least Q1H during first 24 postop hours; then at least Q2H when pt. is in bed; having pt. take 5 slow, relaxed diaphragmatic breaths, then rest for a few min. & holding breath upon inspiration for 3 seconds will increase effectiveness;

— at least Q2H, have pt. cough to loosen & raise mucus, while splinting operative incision with an arm or pillow; forceful, prolonged exhalation can be used to stimulate coughing; direct, external, manual stimulation of the trachea also may trigger the cough reflex; clapping pt.'s back with a cupped hand helps to loosen secretions; record whether cough is productive & pt. has been able to mobilize secretions;

— keep an endotracheal suction machine & sterile equipment at the bedside; when so ordered, employ endotracheal stimulation & suctioning for those unable to bring up tenacious mucus; oxygen should be given before & after procedure; IPPB treatments &/or postural drainage may be indicated; re-breathing $CO_2$ is sometimes used;

— assess condition of lungs by auscultation & percussion; be aware of chest x-ray results;

— do not permit anyone in pt.'s room to smoke, even when $O_2$ is not being used;

— have pt. sit up in high Fowler's (to facilitate thoracic expansion) as soon as condition permits; leg dangling & progressive ambulation should be done as soon as surgeon permits.

Proceed to NCP Guide #2:42, *"General Postoperative Nursing Care, Part B: Support of Cardiovascular, Genitourinary and Gastrointestinal Functions."*

**Recommended References**

"After Surgery: How You Can Avert the Obvious Hazards . . . and the Not-So-Obvious Ones Too," by Edwina McConnell. *Nursing '77,* March 1977:32–38.

"General Postoperative Nursing Care, Parts B & C." NCP Guides #2:42, 2:43, 2nd Ed., Nurseco, 1980.

"General Preoperative Nursing Care." NCP Guide #2:44, 2nd Ed., Nurseco, 1980.

"Safeguarding Your Patient After Anesthesia," by Betty J. Smith. *Nursing '78,* October 1978:53–56.

# General Postoperative Nursing Care, Part B:
## Support of Cardiovascular, Genitourinary, and Gastrointestinal Functions

**Specific Considerations, Potential Patient Outcomes, and Nursing Actions:**

1) Cardiovascular Function

The patient will regain normal cardiac function, circulation, and blood volume; the patient will be free of preventable complications or have them quickly recognized and controlled:

— note preoperative pulse & BP; assess changes in vital signs & report an increasing pulse rate &/or a dropping BP; take apical pulses for one full min. to ensure accuracy;

— note color of nailbeds & lips, note condition of skin; compare with preop description & consider significance of changes; report signs of shock (cyanosis; cold, clammy skin; diaphoresis);

— watch cardiac monitor, if used, for dysrhythmias; take regular arterial pulse pressure & central venous pressure readings; see NCPG #2:40, "CVP Line"; report significant changes;

— review standard procedures for cardiac arrest, shock, serious dysrhythmias; have emergency equipment available; know that early detection & management can prevent serious & permanent damage;

— administer prescribed cardiac medications PRN;

— observe operative incision, dressings, & drainage tubes regularly & as frequently as needed to note early, unusual amts. of bleeding;

— observe & report restlessness & apprehension (bleeding? pain? respiratory distress & hypoxia?), confusion or coma (cerebral anoxia?), yawning (increased $CO_2$?), chest pain (embolus? MI? other?);

— position when possible in a supine, head elevated, slight semi-Fowler's or side-lying position in good body alignment; ask pt. to move legs & flex feet to prevent peripheral pooling of blood;

— avoid changing pt.'s position rapidly or moving pt. suddenly, as circulatory collapse can occur in early postop recovery period when vital signs are still unstable;

— consider pain as a cause of postop hypotension & administer analgesic PRN, watching effects on pt. closely;

— keep pt. warm, but avoid overheating; pt. should neither shiver nor perspire.

2) Fluid & Electrolyte Balance

The patient maintains an optimum fluid and electrolyte balance; the patient is free of imbalances and preventable complications:

— refer to NCPG #3:48 & 3:49, "Fluids & Electrolytes, Part A and Part B";

— accurately monitor & record all fluid intake & output; estimate diaphoresis & wound drainage;

— note color & amt. of urine output; measure & record specific gravity;

— if present, keep nasogastric tube functioning & patent until peristalsis returns & tube is removed; irrigate PRN with measured amt. N/S, subtracting amt. used from returns; record color & amt. gastric drainage;

— measure & record amt. of all other drainage from tubes, describing color & odor; ensure they are kink-free, unclamped & properly functioning;

— administer & monitor parenteral fluids, vitamins/minerals, blood, etc.; refer to NCPG #2:46, "Intravenous Therapy: General Principles";

— observe pt. for adverse infusion reactions (fever, chills, rash, hives, dyspnea, chest pain, hemoptysis, hematuria, etc.); be alert to signs of pulmonary edema (orthopnea, cough, pink sputum, anxiety, rapid pulse); note how much IV fluids were given before & during surgery; keep IV rate no faster than ordered;

— record & report any signs of edema, excessive thirst, urinary output decreasing or below 25 ml./hr., diarrhea, vomiting, muscular contractions or weakness; refer to NCPG #2:48, "Potassium Imbalance";

— give antiemetics PRN as ordered for nausea or vomiting;

— when oral fluids permitted, maintain adequate intake of fresh water & fruit juices;

— weigh pt. daily on same scale, at same time, with same amt. of clothing.

3) Elimination

The patient will be relieved of abdominal distention related to flatus; the patient will resume normal urinary and bowel elimination:

— palpate supra-pubic region for bladder distention; get pt. up to void, if possible, at 3-4 hr. intervals & PRN; if indwelling urethral catheter in place, keep it unkinked & draining without dependent loops to adversely affect gravity flow; refer to NCPG #2:39, "Catheters: Indwelling Urethral";

— discourage pt. from swallowing air via drinking straw or by mouth breathing;

— use colon tube, ambulation or, if permitted, warm baths to relieve flatus; medication may be ordered;

— listen to bowel sounds; note return of peristalsis & passage of flatus;

— if adequate hydration & ambulation is present, administer suppositories, enemas & laxatives as ordered on schedule PRN; note color, odor, amt. & consistency of first bowel movements postop; report diarrhea.

Proceed to NCP Guide #2:43, *"General Postoperative Nursing Care, Part C: Support of Auxiliary Functions."*

**Recommended References**

"Catheters: Indwelling Urethral." NCP Guide #2:39, 2nd Ed., Nurseco, 1980.

"Central Venous Pressure Line." NCP Guide #2:40, 2nd Ed., Nurseco, 1980.

"Fluids & Electrolytes, Part A: Fluids." NCP Guide #3:48, Nurseco, 1977.

"Fluids & Electrolytes, Part B: Electrolytes." NCP Guide #3:49, Nurseco, 1977.

"General Postoperative Nursing Care, Part C: Support of Auxiliary Functions." NCP Guide #2:43, 2nd Ed., Nurseco, 1980.

"Intravenous Therapy: General Principles." NCP Guide #2:46, 2nd Ed., Nurseco, 1980.

"Postoperative Assessment: the Key to Avoiding the Most Common Nursing Mistakes," by Theresa Croushore. *Nursing '79*, April 1979:47–51.

"Potassium Imbalance." NCP Guide #2:48, 2nd Ed., Nurseco, 1980.

"Toward Complication-Free Recoveries for Your Surgical Patients—Part Two," by Edwina A. McConnell. *RN*, July 1980:34–38.

# General Postoperative Nursing Care, Part C:
## Support of Auxiliary Functions
### (Musculoskeletal & Neurological Functions, Infection Control, Safety & Comfort)

**Specific Considerations, Potential Patient Outcomes, and Nursing Actions:**

1) Musculo-
   skeletal
   Function

The patient will resume optimum body functioning, joint mobility and activity; the patient will be free of preventable complications of disuse muscular atrophy, contractures, thrombophlebitis, embolus and nerve injury:
   — maintain correct body alignment at all times, supporting pt. with pillows, pads, foot boards, sand bags & other devices needed to protect pt. & preserve function;
   — massage & protect bony prominences, especially sacrum, hips & heels;
   — keep knee gatch flat; do not permit knees or hips to remain sharply flexed for any period over 10 min.;
   — wrap legs with elastic bandages from toes to groin to promote venous return; re-wrap at least Q8H & PRN when loose;
   — change position regularly & at least Q2H; use gentle, firm support of pt. & operative site when moving; avoid jerkiness & sudden pulls;
   — perform passive & active range of motion exercises as soon as pt. regains consciousness & vital signs are stable; refer to NCPG #1:47, "Range of Motion Exercises";
   — progress slowly from a bedside sitting position, "dangling" legs, to a few steps at the bedside, then to gradually increasing distances & lengths of time, walking or sitting in chair; check pulse & BP before & after getting pt. up;
   — apply a scultetus or straight abdominal binder for support when indicated for comfort, for support of muscles or heavy dressings & for the obese pt.

2) Infection
   Control

The patient will be free of wound and skin infections, upper or lower respiratory infections, phlebitis, thrombosis or other infections:
   — note & report temperature elevations of two or more degrees after the third postop day;
   — administer prophylactic antibiotics as ordered, checking literature & pharmacist for most effective administration;
   — wash hands thoroughly before & after pt. care; use strict aseptic technique when handling IV infusion system, operative site drainage tubes & dressings, indwelling catheters, endotracheal suction catheters, syringes & needles;
   — try to prevent persons with URI or skin infections from visiting or caring for pt.;
   — keep pt.'s bedding clean, dry & free of avoidable contaminants;
   — give regular & complete oral hygiene;

— describe color, odor of all drainage; observe wound site for warmth, redness, purulent drainage; observe IV site for warmth, redness, palpable vein cord; inspect legs for signs of phlebitis; report sudden or unexpected pain in arms, legs, chest or abdomen; observe urine for cloudiness; report pt. complaints of chills, malaise, cough, nasal discharge.

3) Safety, Comfort, & Psychosocial Adjustment

The patient will adapt effectively to trauma of surgery and stress of hospitalization; the patient will verbalize relief of pain and fears; the patient will express a growing confidence with self-care; the patient will be safe from falls, injuries or other untoward incidents:

— keep pt. warm, in a reasonably comfortable position & protected from injuries caused by equipment or supplies, poor lighting, spills on wet floors, etc.; keep bedrails up until pt. fully responsible for own ambulation;

— administer analgesics liberally first 24-72 postop hours, & after that, less often but still when necessary to keep pt. comfortable & able to participate in care; observe for over-sedation (hypoventilation, constipation, disorientation, etc.); refer to NCPG #1:30, "The Patient Experiencing Pain";

— be available to pt./family/friends for expressing of feelings, for asking questions; explain what is happening, how s/he is progressing, & what is expected of pt. to facilitate recovery;

— encourage short, cheerful visits from family & friends, but avoid tiring pt.;

— provide sensory stimulation PRN for pt., orienting to time, date, place; call attention to sights & sounds, news outside the hospital, etc. but avoid excessive noise which produces tension & fatigue & precludes adequate rest; refer to NCPG #1:32, "The Patient Experiencing Sensory Disturbances";

— observe for signs of tension, irritability, restlessness, withdrawal, depression, anger, or other behavioral cues which need assessment for cause; refer to nursing guides for appropriate behaviors; ask pt. what is happening & how things are for the present, identifying feelings & thoughts; examine all reasonable possibilities & seek consultation PRN;

— frightening dreams are common; the pt. often needs to relive overwhelming experience of surgery; give the pt. ample opportunity to talk about his experiences; explain the need & value to family & friends; refer to NCPG #1:30, "Responses to Loss: the Grief and Mourning Process";

— as recovery progresses & the pt. indicates readiness, begin preparations for discharge with pt./family/friend teaching re: diet, medications, activity, care of dressings & incision, community resources, etc.; see NCPG #1:49, "Teaching Patients: General Suggestions," and NCPG #1:50, "Teaching Patients: Specific Plan for Skills and Procedures."

**Recommended References**

"Range of Motion Exercises." NCP Guide #1:47, 2nd Ed., Nurseco, 1980.

"Responses to Loss: the Grief and Mourning Process." NCP Guide #1:31, 2nd Ed., Nurseco, 1980.

"Teaching Patients: General Suggestions." NCP Guide #1:49, 2nd Ed., Nurseco, 1980.

"Teaching Patients: Specific Plan for Skills and Procedures." NCP Guide #1:50, 2nd Ed., Nurseco, 1980.

"The Patient Experiencing Pain." NCP Guide #1:30, 2nd Ed., Nurseco, 1980.

"The Patient Experiencing Sensory Disturbances." NCP Guide #1:32, 2nd Ed., Nurseco, 1980.

# General Preoperative Nursing Care

**LONG TERM GOAL:** The patient will adapt successfully to an uncomplicated surgical and recovery process.

**General Considerations:**
— **Nursing responsibilities** include assessment, care, and teaching designed to shorten the recovery process and to lessen pain, anxiety, and dependence for the patient.
— Provide a cheerful, competent admission procedure that will help the patient and family feel comfortable and optimistic that the hospitalization and care will be satisfactory. Explain all procedures and preoperative preparation to both patient and family. Refer to subject/diagnosis nursing care planning guides for preop measures specific to expected surgical procedure.
— Obtain and complete preanesthetic and preoperative orders; get necessary consent forms signed; secure and check all patient valuables; check and make arrangements for dentures, contact lens, wigs or other cosmetic aids such as false eyelashes and fingernails.

**Specific Considerations, Potential Patient Outcomes, and Nursing Actions:**

1) Assessment    A preoperative data base of the patient's status will be obtained to facilitate accurate postoperative evaluation:
— refer to NCPGs #4:41 "Assessment of Mental Status," 4:47, 48, 49, 50, "Physical Assessment—Part A, B, C & D";
— monitor & record: temperature (oral and rectal), pulse (apical & radial), respiration (note quality), blood pressure (supine and sitting) & weight (hospital gown, no shoes);
— observe & record color & condition of nailbeds & skin; note areas of redness, rashes, lesions, abnormalities;
— note level of consciousness & orientation, clarity of speech, language difficulties, speech or hearing deficits (and aids);
— check whether right or left-handed; note location & extent of any weakness or paralysis;
— note allergies, any drugs or medications taken in the past 24 hours, any presence of cough, sniffles, or illness other than operative diagnosis; note history of smoking and how much; presence of pacemaker.

2) Psychological/    The patient/family will realistically adapt to the traumatic event and outcome of surgery; the patient/family will demonstrate a
    Emotional    positive, cooperative attitude and behavior; the patient/family will be relaxed and confident, coping effectively with normal
    Care    levels of expected anxiety:
— know that a pt.'s fears of the unknown, of pain, of death, of mutilation or destruction of body image & of separation from the normal environment are common & can be reduced by talking it out with supportive information provided by a health professional;

— question pt. & observe behavior to determine *level* of anxiety & its appropriateness to the seriousness of operation: pt. exhibits joking behavior or appears unaware or unconcerned with prospective surgery & risk (low level anxiety); occasionally worries or expresses some legitimate concerns re: surgery, pain, complications, etc. (moderate level); or pt. is highly restless & unable to be reassured (high level); refer to NCPG #1:22, "The Patient Experiencing Anxiety";

— if the surgery will result in loss of a body part, determine the pt.'s realization & acceptance of this fact; refer to NCPG #1:31, "Responses to Loss . . .";

— learn if pt. has talked to someone who has had similar surgery & how it affects his beliefs & attitudes about his own operation; try to correct misconceptions, reinforce positive attitudes, but beware of giving false or inappropriate assurance;

— arrange for a visit from the hospital chaplain, if pt. so wishes.

3) Physical Care    The patient's body systems are prepared for surgery to assure a safe, uncomplicated operative and postoperative period:

— arrange for appropriate cleansing & preparation of operative site, according to hospital procedure;

— plan for necessary restriction of food & fluids as ordered;

— check & care for elimination requirements, i.e. preop voiding or indwelling catheter; rectal suppository, laxatives, or cleansing enemas;

— tape wedding ring in place; cover head according to your hospital procedure if needed;

— administer preoperative medications as scheduled.

4) Patient/ Family Teaching    The patient will participate confidently in the recovery process as a result of having adequate knowledge; the family will demonstrate application of knowledge in the assistance of the patient's recovery:

— discover what the pt. wants & needs to know re: operation & recovery period (e.g. "How soon can I get up after surgery?", "Will I have much pain?");

— explain & have pt. demonstrate correct turning, coughing, splinting the incision, deep breathing, feet and leg exercises;

— explain what pt. may expect postop, e.g. presence of special dressings, drainage tubes, IVs, monitoring equipment, etc. which will be used;

— reinforce what anesthesiologist and surgeon have told pt., clarifying PRN;

— explain preop medication & its expected effects;

— describe postop course, e.g. time in recovery room, ICU, return to home unit, etc.; have IPPB treatment demonstrated when its use is anticipated.

**Recommended References**

"Assessment of Mental Satus." NCP Guide #4:41, Nurseco, 1978.

"How to Give a Safe and Successful Cleansing Enema," by Mildred Hogstel. *American Journal of Nursing*, May 1977:816, 817.

"Including the Family in Preoperative Teaching," by Marcia Dziurbejko and Judith Larkin. *American Journal of Nursing*, November 1978:1892–1894.

"Is That Pre-Op Patient Terrified?" by Donna Hewitt. *RN*, September 1979:44–47.

"Physical Assessment, Parts A, B, C, D." NCP Guides #4:47, 48, 49, 50, Nurseco, 1978.

"Responses to Loss: the Grief and Mourning Process." NCP Guide #1:31, 2nd Ed., Nurseco, 1980.

"The Patient Experiencing Anxiety." NCP Guide #1:22, 2nd Ed., Nurseco, 1980.

"What Priority Do You Give Preop Teaching?", by Mary Lou Lyons. *Nursing '77*, January 1977:12–14.

# Hazards of Immobility

"Look at the patient lying in bed . . .
the blood clotting in his veins,
the lime draining from his bones,
the scybala stacking up in his colon,
the flesh rotting from his seat,
the urine leaking from his distended bladder, and
the spirit evaporating from his soul."

Asher, Richard A.J., M.R.C.P. "The Dangers of Going to Bed."
*California's Health,* October 15, 1958.

**General Considerations:**
— **High risk patients** are those on bed rest, those who are elderly, obese, acutely ill, recovering from surgery or who have a chronic disease or disability. Physical complications can arise after only 2 days of immobilization.
— Loss of mobility can trigger behavioral responses that are not part of the patient's usual way of functioning and that complicate nursing care (see NCPG Set 1, Section B: "Patient Behaviors").
— Conscientious and comprehensive nursing care plays the key role in preventing complications of immobility.

**Specific Considerations, Potential Patient Outcomes, and Nursing Actions:**

1) Pulmonary Function

The patient will be free of congestion, atelectasis, hypostatic pneumonia, and $O_2$–$CO_2$ imbalance:
— turn, cough & have pt. take 5 deep breaths (holding on inspiration for 3 sec.) Q 1-2H during day, in order to expand lungs & raise bronchial secretions;
— have pt. use a re-breathing tube, blow bottles, or balloons to stimulate deep breathing & adequate $O_2$–$CO_2$ exchange;
— position pt. properly to facilitate ventilation; IPPB & inhalation therapy may be needed;
— observe for elevated temp & pulse, often the first signs of problems; report chest pain, productive cough, signs of URI.

**2) Cardiovascular Function**

The patient will maintain adequate circulation; will do exercises to prevent venous stasis:

— apply elastic stockings/bandages: remove for 10 mins. BID; inspect skin for irritations, tenderness (venous stasis is the most important predisposing factor to phlebitis);

— provide active or passive ROM exercises QD (NCPG #1:47); obtain written permission from Dr. for isometric or muscle-setting exercises;

— have pt. wiggle toes, move ankles & legs at least 5 times Q1H;

— avoid prolonged pressure on a vein (as from knee gatches, bed rolls, dangling, chair sitting, crossing knees);

— observe daily for pain in calf and pedal edema; elevate arms & legs to promote venous return;

— ensure an adequate fluid intake to prevent blood concentration;

— check BP BID.

**3) Skin Integrity**

The patient will maintain skin integrity; will be free of new decubiti:

— know that prolonged pressure can cause any skin to break down; if the pt. is cachexic, the risk is raised accordingly; use sheepskins, water or alternating pressure mattress;

— keep skin dry; wash with warm water & mild soap QD; use massages & emollient lotions to stimulate circulation, particularly over bony prominences & pressure points, then pad PRN; keep bottom sheet dry & free of wrinkles; use old, soft, unstarched bed linens;

— turn Q1-2 H; observe for sacral edema, often the first sign of skin breakdown;

— ensure an adequate food intake high in protein, iron, & vitamins to keep skin in a healthy state;

— read NCPG #4:42, "Decubitus Ulcer Care."

**4) Musculo-skeletal Function**

The patient will maintain joint mobility and good body alignment; will be free of wrist- and footdrop, muscle atrophy/spasm/contractures, external rotation of hip:

— provide a firm mattress, overhead trapeze;

— provide a foot board to keep feet at right angles when pt. in supine position; do not allow weight of bed clothes to force feet into plantar flexion; use a bed cradle;

— adjust bed to ensure an even distribution of pressure on undersurface of leg (prevents muscle spasm); change pt.'s position at least Q2H;

— when pt. lying on back, place trochanter rolls under edge of Q hip, extending from crest of ilium to mid-thigh;

— active or passive ROM exercises at least QD for all joints (prevents joint fluid from solidifying, leading to stiffness);
— provide weight-bearing on legs & feet via tilt table or standup exercises (to retard demineralization of bones);
— consider need for and recommendations of a PT consultant;
— position patient properly:
   • *when in supine position:* the *head* is in line with the spine; *trunk* is positioned so that flexion of hip is minimized; *arms* are flexed at elbow with *hands* resting against lateral abdomen; *fingers* functional or holding a rolled washcloth; *legs* are extended with a small firm support under the popliteal area; *heels* are suspended in a space between the mattress & the footboard; *toes* are pointed straight up; small trochanger rolls are placed under the *hip joint* area; a small folded towel is placed under *small of back* (lumbar region).
   • *when in a side-lying position:* the *head* is in line with spine; *body* is in alignment and not twisted; *uppermost hip joint* is slightly forward & supported by a pillow in a position of slight abduction; *upper arm* is flexed at elbow & shoulder & supported by a pillow; *upper leg* is slightly flexed at hip & knee and supported by a pillow.
   • *when in a prone position: head* is turned to the side and in alignment with the rest of the body; *arms* are abducted & externally rotated at shoulder joint, with light pads under shoulders PRN; *toes* are suspended over edge of mattress; a small, flat support is under the *pelvis,* from the level of umbilicus to upper thigh.

5) Gastro-
intestinal
Function

The patient will maintain adequate patterns of food intake and elimination:
— stimulate pt.'s appetite & food interests by using his favorite foods; permit family to bring in some foods; consider offering a small glass of wine 30 mins. AC;
— wheel pt. to dining room or get up in chair for at least 2 meals/day; provide an attractive tray, pleasant environment;
— offer fluids between meals & small frequent feedings; provide foods high in roughage;
— have pt. use bedside commode if at all possible; provide a regular bowel routine; see NCPG #2:04, "Bowel Retraining."

6) Genitourinary
Function

The patient will maintain an adequate urinary output; will adhere to regimen designed to prevent formation of calculi:
— know that retention & incontinence are usually caused by lack of opportunity to empty bladder completely; have pt. stand or use bedside commode to urinate, if at all possible;
— ensure a fluid intake of 2500cc's/day, unless contraindicated; include cranberry juice to acidify urine;
— refer to NCPG #2:03, "Bladder Retraining";
— observe & chart daily: urine color, amount, frequency, turbidity, specific gravity, & pH.

7) Psychosocial
Function

The patient will be oriented to reality X 3; will be able to cope realistically with current situation:
— spread stimuli out over the day, providing adequate rest periods in-between treatments, meals, other activities; watch for fatigue from too many visitors; provide private room, if possible;
— change the environment by moving bed around in room; move pt. to new room; move pt. (& bed PRN) out of room for periods QD; provide stimuli such as clock, calendar, radio, TV, visitors, roommate; have family bring in some of pt.'s personal possessions; see NCPG #1:32, "Sensory Disturbances";
— have pt. make decisions re: daily care, meals, activities; provide occupational & recreational therapy with whatever means you have available; participation in an active, regularly-scheduled program will do much to make pt. feel worthwhile;
— spend some time QD sitting with pt., listening to complaints, providing opportunities to talk, etc.;
— refer to NCPGs #1:41, 42, 43, "Effects of Hospitalization, Parts A, B, C."

**Recommended References**

"Decubitus Ulcer Care: Prevention and Treatment." NCP Guide #4:42, Nurseco, 1978.
"Effects of Hospitalization: Part A—Tension-Producing Causes; Part B—Assessment; Part C—Prolonged Confinement." NCP Guides #1:41, 42, 43, 2nd Ed., Nurseco, 1980.
"Patient Behaviors." NCP Guides #1:20–33, 2nd Ed., Nurseco, 1980.
"The Patient for Bladder Retraining." NCP Guide #2:03, 2nd Ed., Nurseco, 1980.
"The Patient for Bowel Retraining." NCP Guide #2:04, 2nd Ed., Nurseco, 1980.
"Range of Motion Exercises." NCP Guide #1:47, 2nd Ed., Nurseco, 1980.
"The Patient Experiencing Sensory Disturbances." NCP Guide #1:32, 2nd Ed., Nurseco, 1980.

# Intravenous Therapy: General Principles

**GOAL:** The patient will have fluid and electrolyte balance restored and maintained; the patient will receive parenteral therapy with nutrients and/ or medications free of preventable complications in safety and comfort.

## General Considerations:

— Review your hospital policy and protocol for IV techniques endorsed and suggested. *Procedures vary* with institution, physician preference, professional training and patient needs. Some techniques are controversial, but actions listed below are recommended by a number of authorities. Refer to references.

— **Equipment** for IV Therapy varies; it is important to know correct usage of each set-up and number of drops per milliliter introduced by drip-meter of a given set. Accurate calculation of ml./min. is more reliable than knowing drops per minute.

— A heparin lock (scalp vein "winged" needle or catheter with an attached resealable latex cap) may be used for intermittent administration of medications and to keep open vein for future use. The "lock" is flushed regularly with heparin to maintain patency.

— Long-term (1-6 wks.) IV therapy may be given via central venous catheters, inserted and sutured in place by specially trained RNs. The catheter position is verified by x−ray and the IV system is maintained with rigid aseptic technique by nurses. Drugs which are irritating to vascular surfaces and hypertonic fluids may be thus delivered into the central vein or right atrium for rapid dilution in a large blood volume.

— At home IV therapy is more common now. The hospital discharge coordinator makes the referral to VNA and obtains written consents from patient and responsible family member. The coordinator arranges for proper equipment and supplies to be sent home with the patient, until a list of supplies can be purchased by the family. The nurse sends the teaching record completed by the staff covering what was taught and how much the family understands. Sometimes the VNA nurse will visit the patient in the hospital to establish a relationship and to gather additional information for planning home care.

— The use of final inline filters is recommended by the National Coordinating Committee on Large Volume Parenterals for patients receiving total parenteral nutrition or additives that are heavily particulated and for patients whose immune response is minimal. When used, filters need to be replaced every 24 hours because endotoxins released by trapped microbes can pass through the filter into the patient's system.

— Some drugs are not compatible in certain solutions. Be certain of admixture compatibility before mixing and administering parenteral fluids. Post admixture compatibility guides (available from pharmacy; also see references) on each nursing unit near IV supplies. Review literature accompanying drug if you are not totally familiar with drug being given. Drugs are sometimes added to IV fluids in the pharmacy. Be sure to check label against written doctor's orders. Medications are not injected directly into IV tubing after the infusion has started unless *specifically* so ordered. Some drugs, known to adsorb to surface of plastic bag or glass bottle must be given via tubing close to the venipuncture site.

**Specific Considerations, Potential Patient Outcomes, and Nursing Actions:**

1) Safety

The patient will be protected from unsafe parenteral fluid administration; the patient will be free of preventable complications caused by professional errors;

— check written orders with bottle labels: correct fluids? correct amount? does it have all the additives ordered?

— check bottle for expiration date & for cracks; check solution for discoloration, turbidity (cloudiness), sediment, particles; check plastic bags for leakage; check tubing for discoloration & stains (replace if noted); listen for the rushing sound or look for bubbles when infusion set is connected to container of solution;

— label containers clearly with pt.'s name, room number, date of preparation & any medication (name, dose) added to solution; number containers in order of desired sequence for administration; keep solutions at room temperature.

2) Insertion & Patient Comfort

The patient will be as comfortable as possible during IV therapy; the patient will understand about infusion and related care; the patient will be relaxed and cooperative:

— explain the purpose of IV therapy, the equipment used, the solutions & medications ordered & the technique to both pt. & family;

— examine pt. & select venipuncture site; avoid joint areas whenever possible; save antecubital fossa for obtaining blood samples & to avoid interfering with arm mobility; examine arms carefully before resorting to feet & ankle veins; avoid legs altogether in pts. with poor circulation; use distal arm veins first, moving further up for subsequent insertion sites; choose veins a little larger than venipuncture needle or catheter;

— shave hair from site PRN;

— using friction & outward circular motion, prep site with antiseptic solution: povidone-iodine or 70% alcohol (if pt. allergic to iodine); allow to dry & do not touch skin, once prepped;

— apply tourniquet 6-8 in. above injection site; do not cut off arterial circulation so check arterial pulse (radial);

— for central venous catheter insertion, wear mask & gloves, position sterile drapes, administer s/c anesthesia;

— insert needle or catheter according to your hospital's procedure & training; usually venipuncture device enters at a 30° angle parallel to vein, bevel up to avoid going through the vein back wall;

— use non-irritating type tape to secure needle or intracath directly over injection site & to discourage entry of microorganisms; place second & third tapes under & over needle hub & tube connection to prevent accidental disconnection & dislodging (also reduces mechanical irritation of vein caused by needle movement); make a U-turn with tubing & tape again to pt.'s arm; fasten excess tubing loosely to bed;

— apply iodophor ointment to insertion site, then a dry sterile dressing;
— stabilize hand or arm of insertion site with a *padded* aluminum or plastic splint, arm board or empty IV tubing box; support arm (or leg) on pillow for comfort & support of circulation; stockinette or kerlix roller gauze is often used to reduce airborne contamination & to protect insertion site with restless, confused or delirious pts.

3) Maintenance    The patient's infusion will flow at desired, calculated rate without interruption:
— calculate rate accurately, then establish, observe & maintain correct rate; average rate is 3-4 ml./min. (approx. 40-60 gtts./min.) but rate may be faster for pts. in hypovolemic shock or severe dehydration, and may be slower for hypertonic solutions or when pt. has circulatory, respiratory or renal problems;
— solution container should be elevated to at least 24" (often 36") above venipuncture site to maintain gravity pressure flow; to increase pressure for proper flow rate, elevate container more;
— check the following to maintain proper flow rate; remedy each PRN:
   (1) *clamp* effectiveness? a second one may be added for reliability;
   (2) *needle* moved so bevel may be against vein wall, interrupting smooth flow? try elevating or depressing needle/catheter, then stabilize with sterile cotton gauze pad & tape; sluggish flow may also be helped by slightly rotating it to move it away from vein wall;
   (3) *patient position* adversely affecting flow rate? change to obtain desired effect;
   (4) final inline *filter* clogged or blocked? replace;
   (5) *tubing* kinked or flattened under tape or pt.? tubing has dependent loop below venipuncture site, adversely affecting gravity flow? correct cause;
   (6) *bottle* empty or improperly airvented? bag defective? replace;
   (7) *venipuncture site* and surrounding area red, warm or blanched, cold? discontinue infusion, notify physician and re-start IV at new site;
— avoid taking risks of embolus or thrombus; do not irrigate infusion system.

4) Prevention of Complications    The patient will be protected from preventable complications: local and systemic infection, infiltration, tissue damage, phlebitis, thrombosis, emboli, allergic reactions, circulatory overload, others:
— know causes, signs & symptoms of above complications; observe & record pt.'s response to IV infusion regularly, notifying Dr. of serious changes; discontinue IV therapy if judgment warrants;

— wash hands thoroughly before handling pt. or IV infusion system;
— measure & record urinary output, appearance & specific gravity;
— observe & report fever, chills, skin eruptions, itching, cyanosis, flushing, dyspnea, coughing, sudden changes in pulse or B/P & alterations in consciousness;
— maintain sterile technique in handling IV site & set-up; change dressing at venipuncture site Q24H, applying iodophor ointment; change final inline filters, "keep-open" solution containers Q24H; change IV tubing Q48H and whenever IV site is changed;
— look for moisture leakage at venipuncture site as glucose & moisture is a media for bacteria growth;
— watch for infiltration at site & surrounding area (blanching, swelling coldness); if in doubt, verify by use of a tourniquet 4-6 in. above site & open tubing clamp; if IV solution continues to run, tissue infiltration is occurring or tubing has become disconnected from needle; discontinue IV, remove needle and restart IV at a new site with new sterile needle & tubing;
— note phlebitis signs (redness, warmth, palpable vein cord); discontinue IV, remove needle or catheter and re-start IV in opposite arm or leg with completely new, sterile set-up; apply warm, moist compresses to suspected phlebitis & notify physician;
— label tubing & tape on dressing with date, hour changed & initial;
— know drugs to be added to IV solution or given IV push; check admixture compatability, recommended dilution, desired rate of absorption, & both expected & untoward reactions to observe & report; check venipuncture site for normalcy, confirm presence of needle/catheter in vein, & be certain procedure conforms correctly with type of drug & type of IV infusion set being used;
— teach pt. & family to note untoward reactions of IV infusion & to report promptly new symptoms and signs.

5) Recording   Documentary evidence of IV therapy will be maintained accurately and completely:
— record date & time infusion started, type of venipuncture device used, type of antibiotic ointment applied, rate, amt. & type of IV solution being infused, name & dosage of any drug, vitamin or mineral added to solution, & time therapy was terminated; sign each entry;
— chart regularly progress of infusion, when parts of system are changed & by whom, appearance of injection site, pt. reaction & any professional actions taken to prevent or control complications.

6) Termination of Therapy — Intravenous system will be removed safely, correctly and with a minimum of discomfort for patient:
   — clamp tubing, remove tape carefully & completely, gently remove protective dressing;
   — remove needle or catheter quickly, holding sterile pad over site & applying direct pressure for 30 seconds, while elevating pt. arm to drain away blood from venipuncture site & helping to prevent a hematoma;
   — apply antibiotic ointment & a band-aid or dry, sterile dressing;
   — assist pt. to change position or get up, if permitted; observe reaction & check pulse & B/P.

**Recommended References**

"Home I.V. Therapy," by Sharon Michael. *American Journal of Nursing*, July 1978:1223–1226.

"Intravenous Therapy—A Special Feature," a series of articles: "How To Insert an I.V.," "Final Inline Filters," "Fundamentals of I.V. Maintenance," "I.V. Drug Incompatibilities," and "Compatibility Guide for Combining I.V. Medications," by various authors. *American Journal of Nursing*, July 1979:1267–1295.

"IV Fluids and Electrolytes: How to Head Off the Risks," by Sara J. White. *RN*, November 1979:60–63.

"Long-Term I.V. Therapy: A New Approach," by Millie Lawson, Joseph Bottino and Kenneth McCredie. *American Journal of Nursing*, June 1979:1100–1103.

"Preventing Incompatibility in I.V. Admixtures." *Nursing '80*, February 1980:48–49.

"Troubles with I.V.'s? Try These Tips and Techniques," by Catherine Manzi and Susan Masoorli. *Nursing '78*, October 1978:78–82.

# Nursing Diagnoses

**Origin:** This list of nursing diagnoses is the result of four National Conferences on the Classification of Nursing Diagnoses.

The goal of the Conferences has been to develop a standard nomenclature of Nursing Diagnoses, comparable to that used by the medical profession.

**WHAT?** Diagnosis is the end product of assessment, and nursing diagnoses refer to those patient needs/problems/concerns that are the *independent* functions of nursing and require nursing intervention.

**WHY?**
- do we need a classification system?
  - to aid development of the nursing profession by focusing on those areas which reflect its unique contribution to health care;
  - to provide a commonly accepted language to aid communication within the profession;
  - to be congruent with many nurse practice acts and the generic Standards of Nursing Practice developed by the ANA, which include the term "nursing diagnosis."

**HOW?**
- can this help the nurse in practice?
  - Specifically, it can help in writing nursing care plans. Oft-asked questions in this area are, "What do we call this problem? How do you write it on the care plan in a few concise words?" This system can help summarize your findings and judgments.
  - When you have done a nursing assessment and identified some patient needs/problems/concerns, go through the list to see if they "fit" into any of the categories. Some of the categories have subsets which more finely define the problem. A further step in refining your diagnosis is to ask yourself: "What is this patient problem related to?"—e.g. depression, related to mastectomy—("related to" is less legally binding than "due to"). The contributing factor will determine the short-term goal or objective for the diagnosis.

This list of nursing diagnoses is an evolving one. Read the recommended references for background information, and watch the nursing journals for new developments. If you wish to know more about the Conferences, write to Clearing House, National Group for Classification of Nursing Diagnosis, St. Louis University, Department of Nursing, 3525 Caroline St., St. Louis, MO 63104.

**NURSING DIAGNOSES:** Accepted*

Airway Clearance, Ineffective
Anxiety, Mild
      Moderate
      Severe
      Panic
Body Fluids, Excess
Bowel Elimination, Alteration in: Constipation
                     Diarrhea
                     Incontinence
Breathing Pattern, Ineffective
Cardiac Output, Alteration in: Decreased
Comfort, Alteration in: Pain
Communication, Impaired Verbal
Coping, Family: Potential for Growth
Coping, Ineffective Family: Compromised
                     Disabling
Coping, Ineffective Individual
Diversional Activity: Deficit
Fear
Fluid Volume Deficit: Actual
                Potential

Gas Exchange, Impaired
Grieving, Anticipatory
      Dysfunctional
Home Maintenance Management, Impaired
Impairment of Significant Others Adjustment to Illness
Injury, Potential for
Knowledge Deficit (specify)
Mobility, Impaired Physical
Noncompliance (specify)
Nutrition, Alterations in:
    Less than Body Requirements
    More than Body Requirements
    Potential for More Than Body Requirements
Parenting, Alterations in: Actual
                Potential
Rape-Trauma Syndrome
Respiratory Dysfunction
Self-Care Deficit (specify level: Feeding, Bathing/Hygiene, Dressing/
                Grooming, Toileting
Self-Concept, Disturbance in:
Sensory/Perceptual Alterations
Sexual Dysfunction
Skin Integrity, Impairment of: Actual
                Potential
Sleep Pattern Disturbance
Spiritual Distress (Distress of the Human Spirit)
Thought Processes, Alterations in

Tissue Perfusion, Alteration in
Urinary Elimination, Alteration in Patterns
Violence, Potential for

Diagnoses "Accepted" but characteristics not yet defined and to be developed:
Cognitive Dissonance
Family Dynamics, Alterations in
Fluid Volume, Alterations in, Excess: Potential for
Memory Deficit
Rest—Activity Pattern, Ineffective
Role Disturbance
Social Isolation

*Reprinted with permission, Clearing House National Group for Classification of Nursing Diagnosis

**Recommended References**
"Nursing Diagnosis: Looking at its Value in the Clinical Area," by Marjory Gordon, Mary Anne Sweeney, Kathleen McKeehan. *The American Journal of Nursing,* April 1980:672–674.
"Nursing Diagnosis: Making a Concept Come Alive," by Mary R. Price. *The American Journal of Nursing*, April 1980:668–671.
"Symposium on the Implementation of Nursing Diagnosis." *Nursing Clinics of North America*. Philadelphia: W.B. Saunders Co., 483–561.

# Potassium Imbalance

**GOAL:** To maintain potassium balance in the body by preventing, or recognizing promptly, hypo- or hyperkalemia.

## General Considerations:

— Potassium (K) is found in intra-cellular and extra-cellular fluids (ICF & ECF). When cellular activity breaks down tissue (catabolic), potassium moves out of the cells, and into the body fluids; when cellular activity builds up tissue (anabolic), it moves into the cells from the body fluids.

— The test done to measure potassium in the body fluids is **serum potassium** (part of serum electrolytes); **normal range is 4.0 - 5.5 mEq/L.** It is virtually impossible to measure the K level within the cells.

— Potassium is poorly conserved by the body: up to 5% of the total body amount is excreted daily, most via urine, remainder via feces. For most people, this daily excretion is made up by potassium present in an adequate diet.

— A normal diet supplies daily K needs mostly via fresh or dried fruits, and high protein foods:

| **Foods high in potassium:** | **Foods low in potassium:** |
| --- | --- |
| • fruits, fresh or dried | • canned fruits |
| • fruit juices, except apple or cranberry | • apple, cranberry juice |
| • high protein foods | • fats |
| • non-starchy vegetables | • carbohydrates |
| • whole grain cereals | • refined cereals |
| • milk solids | |

— Potassium counteracts some of the effects of digitalis on the heart; when serum potassium levels are even mildly reduced, the myocardium becomes more susceptible to the irritability induced by the digitalis. Patients on digitalis or diuretics are usually given oral potassium daily.

— Potassium is absorbed mainly in the small intestine; thus, gastric suctioning, intestinal drainage, repeated vomiting, or diarrhea significantly deplete the body's supply.

— Aldosterone is the hormone most involved in maintaining both potassium and sodium balance in the body; an excess tends to cause Na retention, which can lead to hypokalemia.

— **Nursing responsibilities** include monitoring patient for signs and symptoms of potassium imbalance, prompt reporting and treatment of same, and patient teaching to ensure an understanding of the relationship between adequate nutrition and maintenance of a normal potassium level.

|  | **Hypokalemia** | **Hyperkalemia** |
|---|---|---|

**Common Causes:**

**Hypokalemia**
- inadequate K intake (deficient diet)
- excessive K output (via prolonged diarrhea, vomiting, intestinal drainage, polyuria, gastric suctioning
- any sudden shift of K from ECF to ICF (as in treatment of diabetic acidosis with insulin and glucose)
- seen most often following use of a potent diuretic, or when there has been prolonged vomiting, diarrhea
- usually occurs in combination with some other pathological condition, commonly with congestive heart failure, MI, Laennec's cirrhosis, hypertension, alcoholism, pulmonary edema
- can occur in 3 days in an NPO patient when there is an excess of corticosteroids (as in stress conditions or in Cushing's Syndrome), when there is excessive Na retention (as in edema)

**Hyperkalemia**
- too rapid or excessive administration of IV potassium
- sudden shift of K from intracellular to extracellular fluids (as in newly burned patients where there is a catabolic activity)
- renal failure
- less common than hypokalemia, but more life-threatening, as it may progress rapidly to a dangerous state causing cardiac dysrhythmias and arrest
- often found in patients where cellular activity is breaking down tissue as in new burns, crushing injuries, MI
- commonly occurs in patients with kidney disease, adrenal insufficiency

**Signs and Symptoms:**

**Hypokalemia**
- general malaise and apathy
- decreased tone in skeletal muscles and smooth muscles (ileus, difficulty in voiding)
- muscle cramps
- dizziness on rising, mental confusion
- cardiac dysrhythmias
- serum K level below 4.0 mEq/L

**Hyperkalemia**
- malaise, weakness, muscle flaccidity, listlessness
- mental confusion, irritability
- nausea, diarrhea
- pulse slower than patient's normal
- tingling or numbness in extremities
- serum K level above 5.5 mEq/L

**Treatment:**

**Hypokalemia**
Consists of K replacement, orally via foods high in K or drugs (KCl, Kaon, Potassium Triplex) or IV (KCl):
- usual IV rate of administration of KCl is 40 mEq.Q8H; maximum is 40 mEq.Q2H.

**Hyperkalemia**
- Consists of excreting K from body, often via enemas, colonic irrigations, dialysis

**Nursing
Implications:**

- measure I&O carefully
- provide foods high in K; check with Dr. to correlate with meds. ordered
- refrain from giving enemas (this will only deplete K further)
- monitor lab reports for changes in serum K level
- explain to patient/family what is happening; share positive changes with them

- measure I&O carefully
- ensure careful IV administration
- monitor patient for signs of cardiac dysrhythmias
- monitor lab reports for changes in serum K level
- if patient confused, ensure safety and prevention of falls, etc.
- take & record pulse & respirations accurately & as often as you judge necessary
- explain to patient/family what is happening; share positive changes with them.

# Problem-Oriented Charting

**Definition:**   A logical, systematic approach to assembling and structuring patient records according to patient problems.

**GOAL:**   The patient's problems will be identified, assessed and corrected through the cooperative planning of medical personnel with the patient and family; a reliable, analytically thorough and effective method of documenting patients' health problems and progress will be utilized; patient care auditing will be facilitated via more reliable documentation.

## General Considerations:
— **Idea proposed** by Dr. Lawrence L. Weed in early 1960s; he believed education should enable professional practitioners to be analytically reliable, thorough and efficient rather than to be memory banks. Problem-oriented medical records provide a format consistent with the scientific method of problem-solving.
— **Components** of problem-oriented records include: a data base (medical and nursing history, exam and lab. results); a problem list; initial plans; and progress notes.
— Problem-oriented charting is a natural by-product of the nursing process which incorporates usage of a written nursing care plan. See ANA Standards of Practice and NCPG #1:48, "Steps in Writing a Nursing Care Plan."
— If you are contemplating using this system in your facility, we suggest you thoroughly acquaint yourself with the literature on this subject, attend seminars on Problem-Oriented Charting, talk to others who are using it, and then work with others in your facility to develop policies and procedures needed for smooth implementation and usage.

## Specific Considerations, Potential Patient Outcomes, and Nursing Actions:
1) Data Base    A specific, well-defined body of patient information will be provided for the purpose of determining a patient's health problems:
— obtain a complete nursing history which includes present and past illnesses, health habits & psychosocial data that may affect pt.'s treatment or nursing care; refer to NCPG #4:41, "Assessment of Mental Status," NCPGs #4:47, 48, 49, 50, "Physical Assessment, Parts A, B, C & D," or NCPG #3:19, "The Child: Nursing Assessment Guide";
— refer to NCPG #1:44, "Suggestions for Interviewing," and NCPG #1:46, "RESTORING +—An Assessment Tool";
— know that the "data base" corresponds to the first step of the nursing process: *interviewing and gathering information.*

2) Problem List    Patient health problems relevant to nursing intervention will be identified:
— consider for inclusion: health hazards, allergies, abnormal signs/symptoms, social or behavioral problems, family problems which affect the patient's illness or recovery, and needs for assistance with activities of daily living or health teaching;

— see NCPG #2:46 "Nursing Diagnoses: Tentative List";
— give each problem a date (when identified), a sequential number & a succinct title; compile a list & attach to the front of the chart; have list differentiate between "active/current" problems and "inactive/resolved" problems;
— update & improve definition or statement of problem when more information becomes available;
— when a problem is resolved or redefined, the old problem number is not reused;
— group, if desired, related problems (such as health teaching needs or various aspects of activities of daily living);
— know that the "problem list" corresponds to second step of the nursing process: *identifying the patient's needs/problems/concerns, i.e. the nursing diagnosis.*

3) Initial Plans    A standardized format will be provided that indicates a desired outcome and the methods to be used to achieve this:
— incorporate into the initial plan for each problem, provisions for answering three questions:
(1) What else do I need to know about this problem? (diagnostic tests, further interviewing & observations to be made)
(2) What can I do about resolving the problem now? (specific medical and nursing orders, counseling and care)
(3) What will I tell the patient/family about the plans for solving this problem? (patient/family educational measures)
— the "initial plan" may be written in regular NCP format; see NCPG #1:48; use ink for entries, initial & date them (the nursing care plan of problem oriented chart becomes a permanent record);
— specify clear, measurable & realistic objectives or goals (desired outcomes) for each problem identified;
— state several specific nursing actions/approaches to achieve the desired results or goals; establish priorities of actions, considering therapeutic goals, basic human needs within the context of this unique individual patient, & standards of nursing practice;
— this initial NCP may be written directly on the progress notes or on the Kardex card; if the latter, a notation to this effect must be on the progress notes to ensure a complete record, & the Kardex card must become a part of the chart after discharge;
— know that completion of the "initial plan" corresponds to the third & fourth steps of the nursing process: *specifying goals and objectives & prescribing nursing actions.*

4) Progress Notes    Pertinent changes in the problem's status or increments of progress in the patient's response to the treatment plan will be recorded accurately and clearly:
— progress notes may be charted in one of three forms:

(1) *Flow sheets* (graphic-type sheets) to record acute or chronic problems which have many components, treatments, nursing actions and/or repetitive observations & measurements, e.g. vital signs, neuro checks; (the type of form most satisfactory is probably one you develop to meet specific needs of the unit);

(2) standardized *SOAP* format, to be used for writing progress notes on a problem already identified:

S-ubjective information: what the pt./family *says* about the problem; symptoms, complaints, etc.;

O-bjective information: *professional observations,* lab & X–ray reports, various measurements, vital signs;

A-ssessment of Problem: your interpretation, evaluation of the pt.'s response to care, i.e. has the problem changed? how? (increased, decreased, modified by new factors?);

P-lan for follow-up of Problem: what should be done next?

— a popular suggestion now is to include I-E-R after the S-O-A-P note:

| | |
|---|---|
| I-ntervention or | |
| I-mplementation: | measures accomplished for the pt. to alleviate problem; |
| E-valuation: | how effective was the measure and what was the pt.'s response? |
| R-evision: | how should the care plan now be changed? |

(3) *Narrative Notes:* written summaries of incidents, accidents, temporary problems, or current pt. situations (return from recovery room, weekend pass from hospital, etc.); title these "miscellaneous" notes: "accident" (or whatever), & chart sequentially on the progress notes, including a date, time & signature;

— when do you chart a progress note?

(1) on admission (narrative type);

(2) whenever you wish to record a measurement, etc. (flow sheet);

(3) whenever there is a change in pt. status or condition (SOAP format);

(4) *at least* once a week in acute hospitals, and *at least* once a month in extended care facilities (narrative or SOAP type);

(5) whenever the pt. is transferred to another unit, health facility, or is discharged (narrative type).

— write all progress notes on the same progress sheet in timed sequence; give date, time, problem number & title;

— when problems are resolved, so state under the "P" of SOAP and mark it "resolved" on the problem list with the date & your name;

— if the problem is not resolved, but you are changing some aspect of the nursing approach, so state under "P" of SOAP note & change it on the Kardex care plan with the date & your name/initials;

— know that the assessment/evaluation of the pt.'s problems & revision of the plan as needed correspond to the fifth & sixth steps of the nursing process: *implementing nursing actions and evaluating patient response to care;*

— upon discharge or transfer, all problems, current & resolved, are reviewed & summarized by the physician, nurse & other professionals who have identified problems for that pt.; a separate chart form is usually provided for this purpose, or it may be recorded on the progress notes; if pt. is being transferred to a convalescent hospital, rehabilitation center or nursing home, make sure a copy of the discharge summary is sent; include data which will be most helpful to the health care staff; provide a copy of the instruction sheet(s) given to pt. & family along with a summary of the educational outcomes that were achieved.

**Recommended References**

"A Visiting Nurse in a Problem-Oriented Group Practice," by Martha Reines. *American Journal of Nursing,* July 1979:1225, 1226.

"Assessment of Mental Status." NCP Guide #4:41, Nurseco, 1978.

"Handbook of Problem Orientation for Nurses." Medical Center Hospital of Vermont, Burlington, VT 05401.

"Let's Set the Record Straight," by Mary Reilly. *Nursing '79,* January 1979:56–61.

"Nursing Diagnoses: Tentative List." NCP Guide #2:47, 2nd Ed., Nurseco, 1980.

"Patient-Oriented Recording—A Better System for Ambulatory Settings," by Betty Ansley. *Nursing '75,* August 1975:52, 53.

"Physical Assessment, Parts A, B, C & D." NCP Guides #4:47, 48, 49, 50, Nurseco, 1978.

"Problem-Oriented Record-Uniting the Team for Total Care," by Alice Robinson. *RN,* June 1975:23–28.

"RESTORING +—An Assessment Tool." NCP Guide #1:46, 2nd Ed., Nurseco, 1980.

*Standards for Nursing Practice.* Kansas City, MO: American Nurses' Association

"Steps In Writing Nursing Care Plans." NCP Guide #1:48, 2nd Ed., Nurseco, 1980.

"Suggestions for Interviewing." NCP Guide #1:44, 2nd Ed., Nurseco, 1980.

"The Child: Nursing Assessment Guide." NCP Guide #3:19, Nurseco, 1977.

# Traction: General Principles

**Definition:**   The application of force through a system of ropes, pulleys and weights to an injured or diseased body part in order to immobilize it in a correct position.

**LONG TERM GOAL:**   The patient's affected body part will be maintained in proper alignment, and will be immobilized via traction for rest and healing; the patient will be free of preventable complications related to circulatory and nerve impairment and immobility.

## General Considerations:
— **Methods:** traction may be applied to the skin with tape, bandage or halter; or secondly, directly to the skeletal system with bone wires, pins, or tongs.
— **Types:** traction may be a "running," direct, one plane pull such as "Buck's" extension; or it may be a "floating," indirect, suspension kind such as "Russell's" leg traction.
— **Purposes:** to relieve pain and muscle spasm; to prevent or correct a contracture deformity; to stretch muscles, regaining more normal length and alignment; to immobilize, reduce and provide rest for a fracture.
— Nurses of orthopedic patients need to be expert in applying knowledge of body mechanics, functional body alignment, prevention of circulatory and nerve impairment, preservation of skin integrity and psychosocial adjustment of the confined patient. Refer to appropriate nursing care planning guides PRN.

## Specific Considerations, Potential Patient Outcomes, and Nursing Actions:
1) Maintenance    The patient's traction will be effectively and correctly maintained:
   of Traction     — after consulting with the attending physician on the following points of information, hold a nursing care planning conference with those who will be assigned to the pt.; record pertinent information on the nursing care plan & on a notice at the pt.'s bedside; know . . .
   (a) purpose & working principle of this pt.'s traction;
   (b) correct position of ropes, pulleys, supports (pillows or sandbags, bed elevation) & amt. of weight to be used;
   (c) activities & movement permitted to pt.; and
   (d) type & frequency of observations to be made for nerve function, circulation, alignment, infection & traction effectiveness;

— normally, pt. is placed on a firm mattress with a bedboard, footboard (supports), overhead frame & trapeze; place bedside stand & necessary items within easy reach of pt.; be sure bellcord & phone are also accessible; keep pt. centered in bed, correct alignment with head of bed elevated 30-45°;

— ensure that ropes & pulleys are in straight lines, at correct angles, unobstructed (not resting on bed, floor, or anything to keep from hanging freely as intended) & not easily disturbed; let weights hang free, off the floor & away from the bed; do not remove weights except with explicit written permission of physician; keep slings (when used) clean, dry, secure & providing support without damaging pressure areas; check periodically all pillows & sandbags used to maintain comfort & correct position; cover ends of exposed pins with cork or foam ball to prevent injury; check ropes periodically to be sure knots are tight & ropes are not fraying.

2) Maintenance of Patient's Bio/Psycho/ Social Systems

The patient will be maintained in optimum health within the constraints of traction apparatus and will be free of preventable complications:

— adhere conscientiously to principles of good skin care (i.e. keeping skin clean, dry, free of irritants & pressure sources, giving regular massage, changing position when possible, etc.); refer to NCPG #4:42, "Decubitus Ulcer Care: Prevention and Treatment";

— carefully perform nursing care routine for a pt. confined to bed (i.e. maintenance of optimum nutrition & fluid intake, adequate bowel & bladder function, correct body alignment, regular range of motion exercises, deep breathing exercises, psychosocial stimulation, etc.); refer to NCPG's #1:41, 42, 43, "Effects of Hospitalization: Part A: Tension-Producing Causes, Part B: Assessment and Part C: Prolonged Confinement"; refer to NCPG #1:47, "Range of Motion Exercises," and NCPG #2:45, "Hazards of Immobility";

— include the pt./family in the plan of care & treatment; in addition, teach pt./family what signs & symptoms to note & report promptly; encourage pt. to participate in unit activities & occupational/diversional therapy; be willing and accessible to listen to concerns & feelings.

3) Assessment of Patient Status

Significant parameters relevant to patient's status will be observed, evaluated, documented and reported when necessary to appropriate personnel:

— the following items should be observed and assessed Q1H during the first 24 hrs. after traction is applied, then Q2H for 24 hrs., then Q4H as deemed medically advisable or ordered:

*Traction* parts: position correct? functioning as intended?

*Body Alignment:* functionally neutral, correct position? feet & wrists supports in place? external rotation of limbs being prevented?

*Sensation:* pain in involved part or elsewhere? numbness, tingling, needles & pins prickling, weird or strange feeling? diminished sensation? change in reaction to sharpness of pin pricks on the dorsum of the feet (especially area between great & first toes)?

*Movement:* muscle spasm? loss of ability to move involved part? decrease or loss of dorsiflexion in the affected extremity? diminished ability to flex fingers or toes? hand grip: strong, weak or absent?

*Pressure Points:* presence of pulses in affected extremity? any pressure being exerted on bony prominences, heels, Achilles tendon just above heel, under knees (popliteal space), below knee to side around the head of the fibula (peroneal nerve path), sacrum, or sites where traction or splints & slings touch skin?

*Skin Color:* redness, blanching, cyanosis or mottling of skin? any breaks, abrasions, rashes?

*Skin Temperature:* warm or cool to touch? changes since last observation?

*Skin Condition:* edamatous? dry? diaphoretic? irritated?

*Infection:* pin sites, dry, clear, normal in appearance? venipuncture sites normal? any oozing drainage or odor beneath bandages, casts, or splints? urine clear, amber? lungs clear? temperature elevations?

*Bandages & Dressings:* loose, wrinkled, slipping? need reinforcement?

— record all observations & assessments on a *flow* sheet record form, so that comparisons can be easily made & changes readily noticed; report PRN to physician, pertinent observation re: pt. status & corrective actions taken.

**Recommended References**

"Decubitus Ulcer Care: Prevention and Treatment." NCP Guide #4:42, Nurseco, 1978.

"Effects of Hospitalization, Parts A, B, & C." NCP Guides #1:41, 42, 43, 2nd Ed., Nurseco, 1980.

"Hazards of Immobility." NCP Guide #2:45, 2nd Ed., Nurseco, 1980.

"Mike J.: A Young Man With A Fractured Femur Part 1: Traction," by Margot J. Stillman. *RN,* July 1978:63–73.

"Nursing Care of a Patient in Traction," by Stephen Cohen. *American Journal of Nursing,* October 1979:1771–1798.

"Range of Motion Exercises." NCP Guide #1:47, 2nd Ed., Nurseco, 1980.